Y0-BFY-272

THE JOHNS HOPKINS WHITE PAPERS

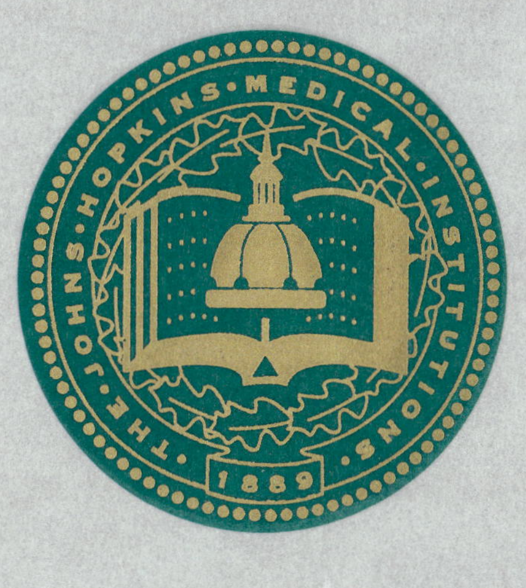

2004

JOHNS HOPKINS MEDICINE
BALTIMORE, MARYLAND

THE JOHNS HOPKINS WHITE PAPERS

2004

JOHNS HOPKINS MEDICINE
BALTIMORE, MARYLAND

HYPERTENSION AND STROKE

Lawrence Appel, M.D.,

Rafael H. Llinas, M.D.,

and

Simeon Margolis, M.D., Ph.D.

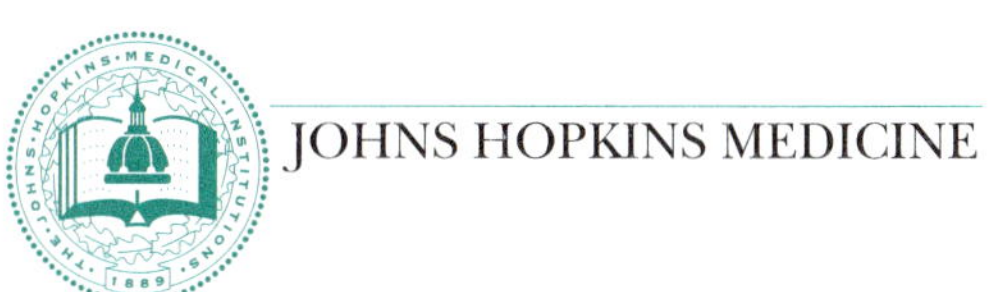

Dear Reader:

You may have moved into a new risk category for high blood pressure without knowing it. Nearly 60 million Americans have hypertension, and guidelines published last year revealed that another 45 million have "prehypertension," putting them at risk for high blood pressure and its complications such as heart attack, stroke, and kidney disease. This White Paper explains the new guidelines in easy-to-understand terms and—drawing on the latest research findings—provides advice on incorporating the recommended lifestyle measures and medications into your daily routine.

One of the greatest risks of hypertension is stroke, which strikes about 700,000 people in the United States each year. Researchers are learning more and more about how to prevent and treat this potentially debilitating disorder, and the most important advances are featured in this White Paper.

Here are some of this year's highlights:

- Find out whether you have **prehypertension**. (pages 9 and 11)
- The **best home blood pressure monitors** for your money. (page 18)
- How to **reduce side effects** from your blood pressure medications. (page 33)
- **Can stress kill?** The link between stress and fatal strokes. (page 43)
- **Cooling therapy**: a promising new treatment for stroke. (page 66)
- How **stroke caregivers** can take advantage of **respite care**. (page 70)

We hope that by learning more about these conditions, you will be able to reduce your blood pressure, lower your risk of stroke and heart disease, and recover more quickly should a stroke occur.

Sincerely,

Lawrence Appel, M.D.
Professor
Departments of Medicine, Epidemiology, and International Health

Rafael H. Llinas, M.D.
Assistant Professor
Department of Neurology

P. S. Don't forget to visit www.HopkinsAfter50.com for the latest news on hypertension and stroke and other information that will complement your Johns Hopkins White Paper.

THE AUTHORS

Lawrence Appel, M.D., received his M.D. from the New York University School of Medicine and performed his residency at Baltimore City Hospital. He is a professor at the Johns Hopkins University School of Medicine, with adjunct appointments in the departments of epidemiology and international health (human nutrition division) of the Johns Hopkins Bloomberg School of Public Health. He is also a practicing internist.

Dr. Appel's clinical research is focused on the prevention of hypertension and cardiovascular and kidney diseases, through both nonpharmacological and pharmacological approaches. He has served on several national policy-making bodies, including the National Heart, Lung, and Blood Institute (NHLBI) Primary Prevention of Hypertension Working Group, the Nutrition Committee of the American Heart Association, and the Institute of Medicine Committee on Evaluation Coverage of Nutrition Services for the Medicare Population.

▪ ▪ ▪

Rafael H. Llinas, M.D., received his B.A. from Washington University in St. Louis and his M.D. from the New York University School of Medicine. He completed his residency in neurology at the Harvard Longwood Program based at the Brigham and Women's Hospital. He also completed a two-year fellowship in cerebrovascular medicine at the Beth Israel Hospital in Boston. Currently he is an assistant professor of neurology and the director of cerebrovascular neurology at the Johns Hopkins Bayview Medical Center. He also serves on the Johns Hopkins acute stroke team.

Dr. Llinas is a member of the American Heart Association stroke division and the Maryland stroke task force. His research interests include neurosonology, diffusion/perfusion imaging, the use of neuroprotective agents, and secondary stroke prevention. He has published articles in such journals as *Stroke, Neurology,* and *Progress in Cardiovascular Diseases.*

▪ ▪ ▪

Simeon Margolis, M.D., Ph.D., received his M.D. and Ph.D. from the Johns Hopkins University School of Medicine and performed his internship and residency at Johns Hopkins Hospital. He is currently a professor of medicine and biological chemistry at the Johns Hopkins University School of Medicine and medical editor of *The Johns Hopkins Medical Letter: Health After 50.* He has served on various committees for the Department of Health, Education, and Welfare, including the National Diabetes Advisory Board and the Arteriosclerosis Specialized Centers of Research Review Committees. In addition, he has acted as a member of the Endocrinology and Metabolism Panel of the U.S. Food and Drug Administration.

A former weekly columnist for *The Baltimore Sun,* Dr. Margolis lectures regularly to medical students, physicians, and the general public on a wide variety of topics, such as the prevention of coronary heart disease, the control of cholesterol levels, the treatment of diabetes, and the use of alternative medicine.

CONTENTS

HYPERTENSION AND STROKE

Hypertension (high blood pressure) is one of the most prevalent disorders in the United States and the most important risk factor for stroke. Stroke is the third leading cause of death in the United States and the leading cause of disability. Because of the close relationship between hypertension and stroke, both topics are addressed in this White Paper.

Hypertension

Hypertension is diagnosed when blood pressure readings are 140/90 mm Hg or above on at least two doctor visits. Nearly 60 million Americans have hypertension, and 9 out of 10 middle-aged people will eventually develop the condition. Although hypertension may not produce symptoms, it is a serious condition and is a primary cause of stroke, coronary heart disease, heart failure, kidney disease, and blindness. Fortunately, in most cases, hypertension is easily detected and usually controllable with lifestyle modifications (such as diet and exercise) and medication.

WHAT IS BLOOD PRESSURE?

Blood pressure is the amount of tension that blood exerts on the walls of blood vessels as it travels through the circulatory system. Blood does not travel through the circulatory system in a steady stream; instead, it is pushed through the blood vessels with every heartbeat. Each time the heart contracts—a period known as *systole*—blood pressure rises as more blood is forced through the arteries. Each systole is followed by a moment of relaxation, or *diastole,* when blood pressure drops as the heart refills with blood and rests before its next contraction.

Thus, pressure in the arteries rises and falls with each heartbeat. For this reason, blood pressure readings include two values: Systolic pressure, the higher number, corresponds with the peak pressure in the arteries when the heart contracts; diastolic pressure, the lower number, reflects the lowest pressure in the arteries as the heart relaxes.

Blood pressure fluctuates throughout the day under the direct influence of three parts of the body: the heart, arteries, and kidneys.

The heart can lower or raise blood pressure by varying the strength of each heartbeat. During exercise, for example, the heart beats faster and more forcefully to raise blood pressure and deliver extra oxygen and nutrients to the muscles. On the other hand, blood pressure drops as the heart slows during sleep. Small arteries are encircled by smooth muscle cells that allow them to expand (dilate) or narrow (constrict). Dilation of these arteries decreases blood pressure, while constriction increases blood pressure. The kidneys affect blood pressure by controlling the volume of blood in the arteries by increasing or decreasing the amount of sodium and water excreted in the urine.

The heart, arteries, and kidneys control blood pressure through an elaborate network of nerves and hormones. Special nerve endings (baroreceptors) in the walls of arteries monitor blood pressure. When pressure increases, the artery walls stretch and the baroreceptors signal the central nervous system to lower the pressure. Blood pressure is similarly monitored in the kidneys, specifically in the glomeruli where blood is filtered.

Three major hormones act in concert to regulate blood pressure: renin, angiotensin, and aldosterone. Renin is an enzyme produced by cells in the kidney; it acts on angiotensinogen, a protein secreted by the liver, to form angiotensin I. As blood flows through the lungs, angiotensin I is transformed into angiotensin II, which raises blood pressure by causing arteries to constrict. (Renin and angiotensinogen are also manufactured in artery walls and other organs, where they constrict blood vessels to control blood pressure locally.)

Angiotensin II also stimulates the release of aldosterone from the adrenal glands, which are located above each kidney. Aldosterone increases blood pressure by signaling the kidneys to retain sodium, which increases both the volume of blood and the amount of blood pumped by the heart. The resulting rise in blood pressure then signals the kidneys to stop secreting renin.

Other hormones also affect blood pressure. Epinephrine (adrenaline) and norepinephrine increase blood pressure in times of stress. Calcitriol (formed from dietary vitamin D) constricts small arteries, while parathyroid hormone dilates them. These two hormones are released in response to changes in the amount of calcium in the blood. However, the exact role of calcitriol and parathyroid hormone in the development of hypertension is unclear.

Atrial natriuretic factor, nitric oxide, and endothelin are additional substances involved in the regulation of blood pressure. Atrial natriuretic factor, produced by the atrium of the heart, causes the

NEW RESEARCH

Rates of Hypertension Increasing

Although the percentage of Americans with hypertension decreased in previous decades, the percentage began to increase at the end of the 20th century.

In a 1999 to 2000 survey of 5,448 adults, nearly 29% (equivalent to 58.4 million Americans) had or were treated for hypertension. This rate was almost 4% higher than that seen in the 1988 to 1994 survey, when about 25% of American adults were estimated to have hypertension. In contrast, between 1960 and 1991, the percentage of Americans with hypertension significantly decreased.

The highest rates of hypertension in 1999 to 2000 occurred in people age 60 and older (65%) and in blacks (34%). Hypertension was also more common in women than men (30% vs. 27%).

About 70% of the people with hypertension in 1999 to 2000 were aware of their high blood pressure and 58% were receiving treatment for it. Hypertension was under control in 53% of those taking antihypertensive medication, but in only 31% of all the survey participants with hypertension.

The percentage of people treated for hypertension and the percentage with their condition under control have improved since the late 1980s. However, people age 60 and older, Mexican Americans, and women had lower rates of hypertension control than younger people, whites, and men.

JOURNAL OF THE AMERICAN MEDICAL ASSOCIATION
Volume 290, page 199
July 9, 2003

The Heart's Role in Blood Pressure

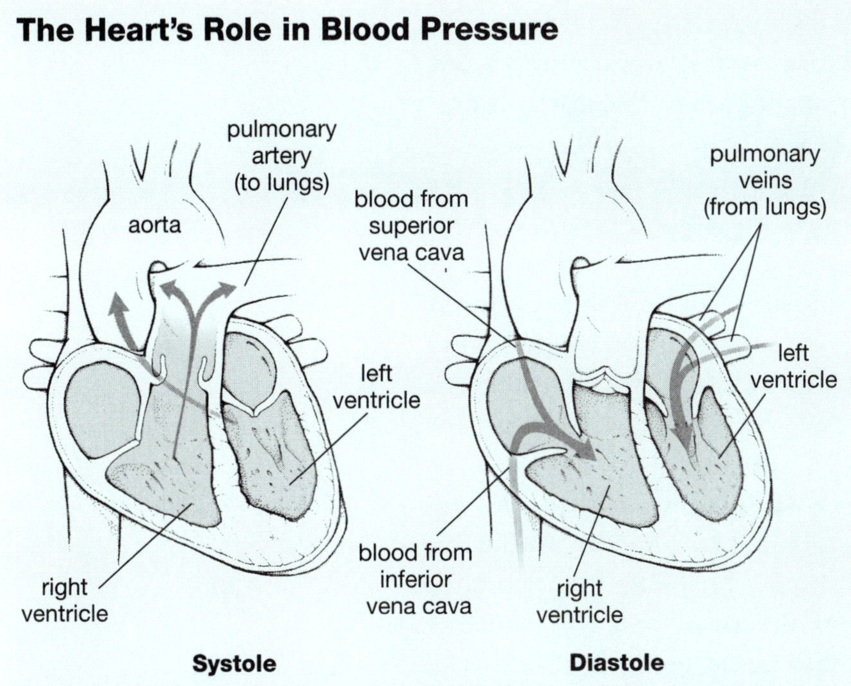

When the heart contracts, blood is pumped by the right ventricle into the lungs and by the left ventricle through the aorta to the rest of the body. The period during which the heart contracts is called systole; the pressure in the arteries during this contraction is called systolic blood pressure. Systolic blood pressure is the higher of the two blood pressure readings.

Diastole is the period during which the heart relaxes between beats and the ventricles fill with blood in preparation for the next contraction. Blood pressure during this time is called diastolic blood pressure.

kidneys to excrete more sodium (and thus more water) and inhibits aldosterone and renin production. Nitric oxide, secreted by the endothelial cells that line blood vessel walls, relaxes smooth muscle cells and causes the arteries to dilate. Endothelin, a hormone released by endothelial cells, causes blood vessels to constrict.

Normally, this complex regulatory system allows blood pressure to rise and fall as needed while staying within a desirable range. In many people, however, abnormalities in this system lead to chronically elevated blood pressure, or hypertension.

CAUSES OF HYPERTENSION

In 90% to 95% of people, it is difficult to pinpoint the exact cause of hypertension. In these individuals, the condition is called primary hypertension. Primary hypertension often results from one or more of the following factors.

Dietary sodium. Diets high in sodium may raise blood pressure in two ways. One, by causing the body to retain water, sodium increases blood volume and thus blood pressure. Two, sodium causes vascular smooth muscle to constrict small blood vessels, which produces a greater resistance to blood flow.

Other dietary factors. Diets low in fruits, vegetables, and dairy products and high in fat and cholesterol raise blood pressure; so do obesity and excessive alcohol intake.

Metabolic syndrome. Researchers have identified a common constellation of abnormalities—obesity, hypertension, high triglyceride levels, low high density lipoprotein (HDL) cholesterol levels, and elevated blood glucose (sugar) levels. The name given to this cluster of health problems is metabolic syndrome.

Obesity, especially a significant accumulation of fat in the abdomen, initiates the abnormalities of this syndrome by producing tissue resistance to the actions of insulin, a hormone that regulates blood levels of glucose. To overcome this resistance, the pancreas increases its production of insulin, and blood levels of insulin rise. Elevated blood insulin levels heighten the activity of the sympathetic nervous system and cause sodium retention by the kidneys—both of which raise blood pressure. For more information on metabolic syndrome, see the feature on pages 6–7.

Genetics. Studies of twins and other members of the same family show that primary hypertension has a genetic component. In addition, researchers have identified a number of genetic mutations that result in inherited forms of hypertension. These mutations, however, account for only a small number of cases of hypertension. Future research may identify additional mutations that are associated with more common forms of hypertension.

Lack of exercise. Physical inactivity can lead to hypertension in several ways. It increases the activity of the sympathetic nervous system, increases the stiffness of the arteries, decreases the release of hormones (such as nitric oxide) that cause arteries to dilate, and reduces the body's sensitivity to insulin.

Secondary Hypertension

When hypertension has an identifiable cause, it is called secondary hypertension. About 5% of people with hypertension fall into this category. Secondary hypertension can be caused by a number of health conditions and medications. It is important to identify secondary causes of hypertension because the resulting high blood pressure can often be cured or controlled by eliminating the underlying problem.

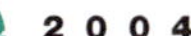

Kidney disorders. Kidney disease that progresses to kidney failure almost always results in hypertension due to the excessive retention of sodium and water in the body. In addition, narrowing of the arteries that supply blood to one or both kidneys, and the resulting reduction in blood flow to the kidneys, causes a form of high blood pressure called renovascular hypertension. In this disorder, the affected kidney senses an inadequate blood supply and secretes excessive amounts of renin, which initiates a chain of events that raises blood pressure. In many people, renovascular hypertension can be cured or controlled by surgical repair of the narrowed arteries.

Adrenal tumors. Three types of adrenal tumors can cause hypertension: primary aldosteronism, Cushing's syndrome, and pheochromocytoma. In primary aldosteronism, overproduction of aldosterone leads to hypertension. In Cushing's syndrome, the tumor secretes excessive amounts of cortisone and related hormones, which raise blood pressure and cause a number of other problems. Treatment of primary aldosteronism and Cushing's syndrome is complicated and does not always lower blood pressure. In pheochromocytoma, the tumor secretes large amounts of epinephrine or norepinephrine, which can cause hypertension. Removal of the tumor may cure the hypertension.

Other hormone problems. Over- or underproduction of thyroid hormone (hyperthyroidism or hypothyroidism, respectively), excessive release of growth hormone by a tumor in the pituitary gland, or increased blood calcium levels due to a tumor in the parathyroid gland can all cause hypertension.

Coarctation of the aorta. In this condition, a portion of the aorta narrows, resulting in hypertension in the upper body and low blood pressure in the abdomen and legs. This disorder, which can be corrected with surgery, is the most common cause of secondary hypertension in young people.

Sleep apnea. People with this disorder stop breathing periodically during sleep. The interruptions in breathing are the result of a temporary blockage of the airway by tissues at the back of the throat. Studies show that people with sleep apnea are more likely to develop hypertension, and the risk rises with the severity of the apnea. Fortunately, treatment of sleep apnea with continuous positive airway pressure, a device that pumps air at high pressure through the nose to keep the airway open, can significantly reduce blood pressure.

Drugs. The following prescription medications can raise blood pressure: corticosteroids such as prednisone (Deltasone and other brands); cyclosporine (Sandimmune, Neoral); tacrolimus (Prograf);

NEW RESEARCH

Smaller Number of Glomeruli Linked to Hypertension

People who have fewer glomeruli are more likely to have hypertension, a study shows. Glomeruli are ball-shaped networks of capillaries in the kidneys that filter blood; their number appears to be determined during fetal development.

The study included 20 white people from Germany, age 35 to 59, who died in motor vehicle accidents. Half of them had primary hypertension, left ventricular hypertrophy, or both. The other 10 had normal blood pressure and were matched to the hypertensive people with respect to weight, height, gender, and age. The investigators removed one kidney from each person during an autopsy and counted the number and volume of glomeruli.

The median number of glomeruli in the hypertensive group was about half that of the group with normal blood pressure (702,379 vs. 1,429,200). However, the average volume of the glomeruli in the hypertensive group was more than twice that of the people with normal blood pressure.

According to an accompanying editorial, glomeruli number can be decreased by low prenatal exposure to protein. Having fewer glomeruli throughout life increases the amount of work each one must do, possibly leading to kidney damage over time and, in turn, an increased risk of hypertension.

THE NEW ENGLAND JOURNAL OF MEDICINE
Volume 348, pages 99 and 101
January 9, 2003

Metabolic Syndrome: A Cluster of Related Problems

Most people have never heard of this surprisingly common condition in which high blood pressure plays a role.

For many years, physicians have recognized that elevated blood glucose levels, high blood pressure, obesity, and abnormal blood lipid levels tend to occur together in certain individuals. This cluster of symptoms—previously called the Deadly Quartet, syndrome X, or insulin resistance syndrome—is now commonly referred to as metabolic syndrome. Almost one in four American adults has metabolic syndrome, which increases the risk of diabetes, coronary heart disease, and stroke.

Diagnosis and Prevalence

In 2001, the National Cholesterol Education Program (sponsored by the National Heart, Lung, and Blood Institute) proposed the following criteria for the diagnosis of metabolic syndrome. A person needs to have at least three of the following five factors to be diagnosed with the condition:

- abdominal obesity (a waist circumference greater than 40 inches in men or 35 inches in women);
- triglyceride levels of 150 mg/dL or greater;
- high density lipoprotein (HDL) cholesterol levels of less than 40 mg/dL in men or 50 mg/dL in women;
- blood pressures of 130/85 mm Hg or higher, or taking an antihypertensive medication; and
- fasting blood glucose (sugar) levels of 110 mg/dL or greater.

While only 7% of men and women age 20 to 29 meet this definition of metabolic syndrome, the percentage rises to more than 40% of those age 60 and older. The condition is more common in Mexican Americans (32%) than in whites (24%) or blacks (22%).

Causes

Virtually all people with metabolic syndrome have insulin resistance, a decreased ability of the body's tissues to respond to insulin. Insulin enables cells to take up glucose from the blood for use as a source of energy. In an insulin-resistant person, cells do not respond adequately to the effects of insulin, and insufficient amounts of glucose enter the cells. As a result, the pancreas produces more insulin to help glucose move into the cells, and blood insulin levels rise. Eventually, the pancreas can no longer produce enough insulin to compensate for the insulin resistance, blood glucose levels rise, and diabetes develops.

Even before the onset of diabetes, however, people may have elevated blood pressure. In addition, increased production of triglycerides by the liver can lead to abnormalities in blood lipid levels, including high triglycerides, low levels of HDL cholesterol, and increased levels of small, dense low density lipoprotein (LDL), which is more likely to cause blood clots than less dense LDL.

Exactly what causes insulin resistance is unclear. However, researchers do know that genetic factors, obesity, physical inactivity, diet, cigarette smoking, and older age each contribute to insulin resistance and therefore to metabolic syndrome. Other factors that make a person more likely to develop insulin resistance include a family history of diabetes in a first-degree relative (a parent or sibling), a personal history of gestational diabetes (diabetes during pregnancy), or polycystic ovary syn-

epoetin (Epogen, Procrit); and nonsteroidal inflammatory drugs (NSAIDs) such as indomethacin (Indocin), celecoxib (Celebrex) and rofecoxib (Vioxx). Some over-the-counter remedies can also elevate blood pressure. These include pain relievers like ibuprofen (Advil, Motrin) and naproxen (Aleve), nasal decongestants, and dietary supplements and weight loss products containing ephedra (ma huang). Illegal drugs such as cocaine and amphetamines can increase blood pressure as well.

SYMPTOMS AND SIGNS OF HYPERTENSION

Most people with hypertension experience no symptoms, and as a result the condition may go undetected for many years. Some individuals complain of symptoms, such as headaches, but most often

drome (a condition characterized by infrequent or absent menstruation, infertility, and excessive body hair).

Complications

Metabolic syndrome increases the risk of numerous complications. Because of its association with insulin resistance, people with metabolic syndrome are more likely to have type 2 diabetes. In turn, diabetes increases the risk of vision problems, kidney dysfunction, nerve problems, coronary heart disease, and stroke.

High blood pressure, high triglyceride levels, and low HDL cholesterol levels are all risk factors for atherosclerosis. Elevated insulin levels are also associated with an increased tendency for blood clot formation. As a result, people with metabolic syndrome have a greater incidence of all types of cardiovascular disease (including nonfatal and fatal heart attacks and strokes) and are at increased risk for premature death from any cause.

Treatment

Treatment of metabolic syndrome focuses on overcoming insulin resistance and correcting any associated abnormalities. The first step in treatment is lifestyle changes. The most important lifestyle change is weight loss through increased physical activity, decreased intake of calories (particularly simple carbohydrates), and increased fiber intake.

Physical activity aids in weight loss, improves responsiveness to insulin, increases HDL cholesterol levels, and decreases blood pressure. An increase in activity need not be dramatic to achieve significant health benefits—even a half hour of brisk walking most days of the week will help.

Weight loss improves insulin sensitivity, reduces insulin levels, and lowers the risk of developing type 2 diabetes. While reduced insulin resistance can occur with as little as a 5-lb. weight loss, better results are achieved with more weight loss. A diet rich in fiber-containing foods—such as fruits, vegetables, and whole grains—can help overcome insulin resistance. Smoking cessation can lessen insulin resistance and help to raise HDL cholesterol levels.

If lifestyle modifications do not correct the associated cardiovascular risk factors, medications can lower blood pressure and improve lipid levels. Thiazide diuretics are considered first-choice therapy for hypertension because they prevent heart attacks and strokes. ACE inhibitors are also a good choice for those with metabolic syndrome because they may reduce the risk of developing type 2 diabetes, in addition to lowering blood pressure. Some people with metabolic syndrome may require statins, which lower LDL cholesterol and raise HDL cholesterol. Niacin, gemfibrozil (Lopid), and fenofibrate (Lofibra, Tricor) can also raise HDL cholesterol and lower triglyceride levels.

Metformin (Glucophage) and the thiazolidinediones pioglitazone (Actos) and rosiglitazone (Avandia) are currently used to treat insulin resistance in people with type 2 diabetes. In addition, according to a 2002 study in *The New England Journal of Medicine,* people at high risk for diabetes (those who are overweight and have elevated blood glucose levels) can prevent or delay the development of diabetes with lifestyle changes and, less markedly, with metformin. However, it is not yet clear whether these medications should be used to treat the insulin resistance that leads to metabolic syndrome.

hypertension is discovered during a routine physical examination or, less commonly, when a patient experiences one of the complications of hypertension: transient ischemic attack (TIA), stroke, visual abnormalities, angina, heart attack, heart failure, intermittent claudication (pain in the leg muscles associated with physical exertion), or symptoms of kidney disease.

Another situation in which people may experience symptoms from hypertension is a hypertensive crisis. In a hypertensive crisis, blood pressure reaches very high levels (diastolic pressures above 120 mm Hg). This condition occurs in about 1% of people with hypertension—usually around age 40—and may be precipitated by an abrupt cessation of antihypertensive medication. There are two types of hypertensive crisis: hypertensive emergency (also called malignant hypertension) and hypertensive urgency.

A hypertensive emergency is accompanied by one or more symptoms that indicate major damage is occurring to the body's organs. These symptoms include chest pain, shortness of breath, seizures, back pain, headache with confusion and blurred vision, nausea, vomiting, and unresponsiveness. When a hypertensive emergency is suspected, people should not eat or drink anything and should lie down until they can be driven to the hospital or an ambulance arrives.

The more common form of hypertensive crisis—hypertensive urgency—is not accompanied by symptoms indicative of major organ damage. Instead, headache and nosebleed are the two most common symptoms. Although this condition requires medical attention, treatment is not needed immediately. However, within a few hours of no treatment, a hypertensive urgency could become a hypertensive emergency.

CLASSIFYING BLOOD PRESSURE

Blood pressure levels used to be classified as optimal, normal, high-normal, and hypertension (stage 1, stage 2, and stage 3). But with the publication of the Seventh Report of the Joint National Committee on Prevention, Detection, Evaluation, and Treatment of High Blood Pressure—more commonly known as JNC 7—a new system of classifying blood pressure was adopted in May 2003. This classification system has three categories: normal, prehypertension, and hypertension (stage 1 and stage 2).

People who used to have optimal blood pressure (less than 120/80 mm Hg) are now considered to have normal blood pressure. The old categories of normal and high-normal blood pressure have been collapsed into a single category called prehypertension (blood pressure levels between 120 and 139 mm Hg systolic or 80 and 89 mm Hg diastolic). As before, hypertension is a blood pressure reading of 140/90 mm Hg or higher. (To find out which category your blood pressure falls into, consult the table at right.)

About one in five Americans has prehypertension. These individuals are at increased risk for developing hypertension and hypertension complications such as heart attacks and strokes. For more information on prehypertension, see the feature on page 11.

Systolic vs. Diastolic Pressure

Historically, doctors have focused on diastolic blood pressure for the diagnosis and treatment of hypertension. But systolic blood pressure

New Guidelines for Evaluating and Managing Blood Pressure Levels

Updated blood pressure guidelines from the Joint National Committee on Prevention, Detection, Evaluation, and Treatment of High Blood Pressure were published in May 2003 in the *Journal of the American Medical Association*. The guidelines, called JNC 7, are summarized in the table below.

To determine your blood pressure category, average your blood pressure readings from at least two doctor visits. If your systolic and diastolic blood pressures fall into different categories, use the more elevated reading. For example, an average reading of 165 mm Hg systolic and 95 mm Hg diastolic means that you have stage 2—rather than stage 1—hypertension.

Lifestyle measures to keep blood pressure under control are recommended for all people—even those with normal blood pressure and those taking medication to manage their hypertension. Lifestyle measures include losing weight if necessary, following the Dietary Approaches to Stop Hypertension (DASH) diet, reducing sodium intake, increasing physical activity, moderating alcohol consumption, and quitting smoking (see pages 20–22).

Blood Pressure Category	Systolic Blood Pressure (mm Hg)	Diastolic Blood Pressure (mm Hg)	What To Do
Normal	<120	<80	Lifestyle measures encouraged.
Prehypertension	120–139	80–89	Lifestyle measures only. If you have diabetes or kidney disease, you may need to take medication to lower your blood pressure to less than 130/80 mm Hg.
Stage 1 hypertension	140–159	90–99	Lifestyle measures. Blood pressure medication is also required—usually a thiazide diuretic. Other types of blood pressure medication may be considered if you have heart disease, diabetes, or kidney problems or if you have had a stroke.
Stage 2 hypertension	≥160	≥100	Lifestyle measures. Also, two blood pressure medications are typically required—usually a thiazide diuretic in combination with an ACE inhibitor, angiotensin II receptor blocker, beta-blocker, or calcium channel blocker. Other combinations of blood pressure medications may be used if you have heart disease, diabetes, or kidney problems or if you have had a stroke.

appears to be a more important determinant of blood pressure-related complications than diastolic blood pressure, particularly in people older than age 50.

In contrast to diastolic blood pressure, which tends to rise until about age 55 and then begins to fall, systolic blood pressure continues to rise with age. Previously, such elevations were thought to be a normal part of aging—caused by a gradual loss of elasticity in the arterial walls. Now, however, a substantial body of evidence shows that high systolic blood pressure with a diastolic blood pressure under 90 mm Hg carries a high risk of heart attacks and strokes. In light of such findings, the new JNC 7 guidelines recommend using systolic blood pressure as the standard measure for the evaluation and treatment of hypertension, especially for people age 50 and older.

The JNC 7 guidelines also recommend that most people with hypertension aim to keep their blood pressure below 140/90 mm Hg, regardless of their age. In people with diabetes or kidney disease, blood pressure should be maintained below 130/80 mm Hg.

Isolated Systolic Hypertension

A high systolic blood pressure with a normal diastolic pressure is common in older adults. In fact, 65% of people over age 60 with hypertension have a condition called isolated systolic hypertension, defined as a systolic blood pressure of 140 mm Hg or higher and a diastolic blood pressure under 90 mm Hg. Isolated systolic hypertension is associated with an increased risk of strokes, coronary heart disease, and kidney disease.

Pulse Pressure

Another possible predictor of blood pressure-related complications is pulse pressure—the difference between the systolic and diastolic blood pressures. Pulse pressure reflects the stiffness of the arteries, and it may be just as important as blockages in the coronary arteries for determining the risk of a heart attack.

Researchers recently pooled the results of three major hypertension studies involving nearly 8,000 patients. They found that the higher the pulse pressure, the greater the risk of cardiovascular complications (such as heart attacks and strokes) and death from any cause.

White Coat Hypertension

Some people have white coat hypertension—consistently high blood pressure readings that are present only when they are examined by a physician or in a medical environment. Blood pressure measurements are normal when taken at home by the patient or a family member or friend. As many as 20% of people likely have white coat hypertension.

Whether to treat white coat hypertension with antihypertensive medication is controversial. Many (but not all) hypertension

A New Definition of "Normal" Blood Pressure

Find out whether you have "prehypertension," and if so, what you can do to reduce your risk of developing full-blown hypertension.

You've been getting your blood pressure checked regularly, and your readings are consistently below 130/85 mm Hg. According to previous guidelines from the Joint National Committee on Prevention, Detection, Evaluation, and Treatment of High Blood Pressure, which were released in 1997, you had normal blood pressure. Now, according to the committee's newest recommendations, you might fall into a new category called prehypertension. This classification was created to help motivate both doctors and their patients to take important steps to prevent hypertension and to reduce the risk of cardiovascular events, such as heart attacks and strokes.

Blood Pressure Classification: The Old vs. the New

According to the old recommendations, "optimal" blood pressure was a systolic pressure less than 120 mm Hg and a diastolic pressure lower than 80 mm Hg. People with these values now fall into the new "normal" category. The previous categories of "normal" (systolic 120 to 129 mm Hg or diastolic 80 to 84 mm Hg) and "high-normal" (systolic 130 to 139 mm Hg or diastolic 85 to 89 mm Hg) have been combined into the new "prehypertension" category. Therefore, prehypertension is defined as a systolic blood pressure between 120 and 139 mm Hg or a diastolic blood pressure of 80 to 89 mm Hg.

New evidence about the risks associated with elevated blood pressure levels prompted experts to update the old blood pressure classifications. "We have found that damage to the arteries begins at fairly low blood pressure levels—levels previously considered 'normal,'" Aram V. Chobanian, M.D., the committee's chair, said at a press conference at which the guidelines were released. (The guidelines were later published in May 2003 in the *Journal of the American Medical Association*.)

The guidelines point out that the risks of health problems like heart attacks, strokes, heart failure, and kidney disease begin to increase when blood pressure levels rise above 115/75 mm Hg. For people 40 to 69 years of age, for example, every increase of 20 mm Hg in systolic pressure or 10 mm Hg in diastolic pressure above this threshold doubles the risk of dying of a stroke or other cardiovascular event.

What To Do

The new guidelines don't recommend that most people with prehypertension take antihypertensive medication, but they do say that these individuals should use a combination of lifestyle modifications to reduce their blood pressure, prevent the development of hypertension, and lower their risk of cardiovascular events. These modifications include losing weight, adopting a diet that emphasizes fruits and vegetables, restricting sodium intake, exercising, and consuming alcohol only moderately. (See the text on pages 20–22 for more details on these lifestyle modifications.)

Such lifestyle measures are also recommended for people with higher blood pressure levels, including those on medication. Using a combination of lifestyle modifications reduces blood pressure more than using only some of them (see the sidebar on page 20).

Still, certain people with prehypertension should be treated with medication. According to the guidelines, such persons include those with diabetes or chronic kidney disease. These individuals may need medication to reduce their blood pressure to below 130/80 mm Hg.

specialists believe that people with white coat hypertension who do not have other risk factors for cardiovascular disease (such as high cholesterol levels or diabetes) do not need to take medication. Instead, they should adopt lifestyle measures such as eating a healthy diet and exercising regularly. However, the general consensus is that people with white coat hypertension who have organ damage from hypertension (for example, kidney or heart disease) need treatment with medication.

Some people experience the opposite problem to white coat hypertension: Their average daytime blood pressure is high, but it is normal when measured in a medical setting. Such people are unlikely to be treated for high blood pressure and therefore may miss out on the benefits of treatment. People with borderline measurements in the doctor's office (systolic blood pressure 130 to 139 mm Hg or diastolic pressure 85 to 89 mm Hg) are more likely to be diagnosed inaccurately.

COMPLICATIONS OF HYPERTENSION

Hypertension can damage both large and small arteries, leading to disease in the tissues and organs supplied by these damaged blood vessels. The tissues and organs most often affected by hypertension are the brain, heart, kidneys, and eyes. Fortunately, controlling blood pressure can help prevent or slow the progression of many of the complications of hypertension.

Brain. Hypertension accelerates atherosclerosis—the buildup of deposits called plaques within the walls of large arteries. If the plaques partially obstruct blood flow through an artery that leads to the brain (for example, the carotid artery), the result could be a transient ischemic attack (a mini-stroke in which symptoms usually subside within 5 to 20 minutes). If a blood clot forms in a plaque-containing artery, it could completely block blood flow and cause an ischemic stroke.

Hypertension can also weaken arteries, resulting in a sac-like bulge (aneurysm) in the artery's wall. Rupture of an aneurysm in an artery supplying blood to the brain can result in a hemorrhagic stroke.

Evidence is accumulating that hypertension can also have more subtle effects on the brain, causing impairments in mental functions such as memory (see the feature on pages 14–15).

Heart. Atherosclerosis in the coronary arteries, which carry blood to the heart, can lead to a type of chest pain called angina when blood flow to the heart is insufficient. Complete blockage of a coronary artery by a blood clot results in a heart attack.

Atherosclerosis is not the only way hypertension can damage the heart. In people with hypertension, the heart works harder to pump against the higher pressures in the arteries. This excess workload thickens and increases the size of the heart's left ventricle. Called left ventricular hypertrophy, this condition affects 30% of people with hypertension and increases the risk of angina, heart attacks, heart failure, and cardiac arrest.

Kidneys. Hypertension can damage the kidneys in two ways: by promoting atherosclerotic narrowing of the main arteries supplying the kidneys and by damaging the small arteries within the kidneys. Both can lead to progressive loss of kidney function and, eventually, kidney failure. Such kidney damage illustrates the vicious circle of hypertension: High blood pressure can lead to kidney disease and atherosclerosis; kidney disease and atherosclerosis further elevate blood pressure; and higher blood pressure causes further kidney damage.

Eyes. Persistent elevation of blood pressure can also damage the tiny arteries that supply blood to the retina (the light-sensitive layer of nerve tissue that lines the back of the eye), resulting in a condition called hypertensive retinopathy. In the early stages of this disorder, the arteries in the retina thicken and narrow. Eventually, these vessels may develop blockages or begin to leak blood and fluid into the surrounding tissue. In very severe cases, the optic nerve (the nerve that carries visual impulses to the brain) may swell and cause vision loss. Hypertensive retinopathy typically evolves gradually, and many years may pass before people notice any changes in their vision.

PREVENTION OF HYPERTENSION

Prevention of any rise in blood pressure is important because organ damage can begin when pressures exceed 110 mm Hg systolic or 70 mm Hg diastolic—long before hypertension is present. Preventing hypertension also eliminates the need for antihypertensive medications, which have potential side effects and can be costly. In addition, people with hypertension who successfully control their blood pressure with medication have a higher risk of hypertension complications than normotensive individuals with similar blood pressure levels. Hence, for many reasons, it is best to prevent hypertension in the first place.

The keys to preventing hypertension are weight loss, a diet rich in fruits and vegetables and low in sodium, regular physical activity, and moderate alcohol consumption (only for those who drink; abstainers should not begin drinking to reduce their risk of hypertension). Such relatively simple lifestyle modifications can have a considerable impact. In one study, for example, a weight loss of just 10 lbs. decreased the risk of hypertension by 50% in people with a systolic blood pressure between 130 and 139 mm Hg or a diastolic blood pressure between 85 and 89 mm Hg. The benefits of prevention appear to be more substantial when all of the

NEW RESEARCH

High Blood Levels of Lead May Increase Blood Pressure

In middle-aged women, elevated blood lead levels are linked to elevated blood pressure, a group of researchers report. The association between lead and higher diastolic blood pressure was particularly strong after menopause.

The investigators looked at data from 2,165 women, age 40 to 59. Women with the highest blood levels of lead (6.4 micrograms/dL on average) were 1.5 times more likely to have systolic blood pressures higher than 140 mm Hg and 3.4 times more likely to have diastolic blood pressures higher than 90 mm Hg, compared with women with the lowest blood lead levels (1 microgram/dL on average). In postmenopausal women, those with the highest blood lead levels had an eightfold increased risk of diastolic pressures higher than 90 mm Hg, compared with those with the lowest levels.

These results are of particular concern, the researchers write, because the lead levels that appear to increase blood pressure are well below those considered safe by the U.S. government.

As women lose bone mass around the time of menopause and afterward, lead stored in their bones during earlier years may be released into the blood and cause blood lead levels to rise, the researchers say.

JOURNAL OF THE AMERICAN MEDICAL ASSOCIATION
Volume 289, page 1523
March 26, 2003

Blood Pressure and Brain Power

Keeping your blood pressure under control may help prevent a decline in thinking skills.

High blood pressure is a known risk factor for vascular dementia (a condition caused by a series of tiny strokes that impair mental function and memory in older adults). Now a new study provides evidence of another link between high blood pressure and future mental decline. The study found that hypertension may play a role in the development of brain lesions that affect mental function.

Blood Pressure and the Brain

Research on the link between hypertension and mental function has reached contradictory conclusions.

In a 1999 study in the *Journal of the American Medical Association*, researchers examined 3,657 people (age 65 to 102). People with higher blood pressures—a systolic blood pressure of 160 mm Hg or higher or a diastolic blood pressure of 90 mm Hg or higher—made more errors on tests of mental status than those with a systolic pressure between 130 and 139 mm Hg or a diastolic blood pressure between 70 and 79 mm Hg. Surprisingly, however, high blood pressure was not associated with a progressive decline in mental function over a six-year period. In addition, test scores were slightly lower in people with normal blood pressure than in those with borderline hypertension.

The following year, a study in *Hypertension* examined mental function in 107 healthy people with moderately high blood pressure (averaging 164/89 mm Hg) and 116 people without hypertension (averaging 131/74 mm Hg). The average age of the participants in both groups was 76. On average, the group with high blood pressure had 10% slower reaction times on mental tests and was less able to remember words or numbers than the group without hypertension. This study was the first to exclude other possible causes of mental decline, such as strokes, and to focus solely on the effects of hypertension. These findings echoed a 1995 study, which reported that each 10 mm Hg increase in systolic blood pressure is associated with a 9% greater risk of poor mental function.

Most recently, a 2003 study in *Psychology and Aging* suggested that hypertension may be associated with white matter lesions (age-related changes that affect the brain's ability to transmit information). These

recommended lifestyle modifications are adopted (see the sidebar on page 20).

DIAGNOSIS OF HYPERTENSION

Hypertension is discovered most often during a routine visit to the doctor. The instrument used to evaluate blood pressure in a doctor's office is called a sphygmomanometer and typically consists of an inflating bulb, an inflatable cuff, and a mercury column gauge. Blood pressure is measured by wrapping the cuff around the upper arm and determining how much pressure is needed to compress the brachial artery—the major artery in the arm. The amount of pressure needed is equivalent to the height of the mercury in the gauge. Thus, blood pressures are expressed in millimeters of mercury, or mm Hg.

Because of concerns about mercury contamination of the environment, the Environmental Protection Agency is encouraging doctors to switch to aneroid or electronic blood pressure devices that use dial or digital gauges, respectively, to indicate blood pressure levels. Some experts are uneasy about these devices, but when used

changes have been linked to declines in mental function, even in people without dementia. In the study, Scottish researchers tested mental function in 83 people in their late 70s and compared the results with similar tests that the participants took when they were 11 years old. Participants with the most white matter lesions had the greatest declines in mental function over time. In addition, people with hypertension had both a greater number of white matter lesions and a greater decrease in mental function than people with normal blood pressure.

How To Prevent Mental Decline

Clearly, evidence is mounting for a relationship between hypertension and decreased mental function. Exactly how high blood pressure might affect mental abilities, however, is still unknown. For example, mental deterioration may be due to hypertension-induced cerebral arteriosclerosis—hardening of the arteries in the brain that interferes with the delivery of blood (which contains vital oxygen and nutrients) to brain cells. A 1997 study linking hypertension to memory loss in the elderly found that hypertensive people had greater brain atrophy (as assessed by magnetic resonance imaging) than people with normal blood pressure. It seems likely that these two changes in the brain could be the basis of impaired mental function.

Further research is necessary, however, to determine with certainty why and how hypertension and mental function are connected. Eventually, such an understanding could lead to new methods for preventing and treating mental decline in older adults.

In the meantime, some research has shown that treating high blood pressure during middle age helps to protect against mental deterioration in later years. A 2002 review article in the *Journal of Neurological Sciences* concluded that lowering blood pressure with antihypertensive drugs can reduce the risk of impaired mental function, and that calcium channel blockers and ACE inhibitors appear to be more effective than diuretics and beta-blockers for protecting mental function.

More research is also needed to examine the relationship between antihypertensive medication and mental function. Knowledge in this area is lacking because, until 1995, researchers focused on making sure blood pressure medication didn't impair mental function (rather than on whether it could have a protective role). In general, control of blood pressure is the only established way to protect against the various complications related to high blood pressure.

properly they can be as accurate as mercury sphygmomanometers.

Regardless of the type of device used to measure blood pressure, the following steps will help ensure accurate results. People should not smoke or consume caffeine in the 30 minutes prior to having their blood pressure measured. They should be seated and at rest for at least five minutes before the measurement. In addition, the results of two or more readings, taken at least one minute apart, should be averaged. Hypertension is diagnosed when the average blood pressure reading is 140/90 mm Hg or higher on at least two separate doctor visits.

Home Monitoring of Blood Pressure

Home monitoring of blood pressure can be useful in determining the presence of white coat hypertension (see pages 10–11) and can help people with hypertension keep track of the effects of lifestyle modifications and medication on their blood pressure. Two types of devices are available for home measurements: mechanical aneroid monitors and electronic monitors. Both types of monitors need to be checked annually against a standard mercury sphygmomanometer at the doctor's office to ensure continuing accuracy.

Traditionally, the best way to measure blood pressure at home has been with a manually operated aneroid monitor that consists of a cuff, bulb, and dial gauge to register blood pressure levels. A stethoscope is also required (most monitors come with one). Advantages of aneroid monitors are their accuracy, consistency, and low price ($20 to $30). Users of aneroid monitors must be able to rapidly squeeze the bulb to inflate the cuff, hear the thumping sounds of blood flow with the stethoscope, read the gauge that records the pressure, and loosen a valve to let out the air slowly. Thus, individuals with hearing or vision problems or limited hand movement (from arthritis, for example) may not be able to use an aneroid monitor.

Electronic home monitors are improving and growing in popularity. Some types have a cuff that inflates automatically; those with manually inflated cuffs will deflate automatically. You need only record the numbers that appear on the digital screen. Electronic monitors are more expensive than aneroid monitors; those with automatic cuff inflation are the most expensive. Prices for electronic monitors range from about $35 to $125. For more information on electronic home monitors and advice on choosing one, see the feature on pages 18–19.

Ambulatory Blood Pressure Monitoring

Ambulatory blood pressure monitors automatically measure and record blood pressures over a 24- to 48-hour period. Such measurements may be useful in the diagnosis of white coat hypertension (see pages 10–11). There is also some evidence that ambulatory monitoring may be helpful in identifying people with drug-resistant hypertension, hypotension caused by blood pressure medication, episodic hypertension, or borderline hypertension (systolic blood pressure 130 to 139 mm Hg or diastolic pressure 85 to 89 mm Hg). Ambulatory monitoring is not necessary when multiple blood pressure readings at the doctor's office are well beyond the threshold for treatment (above 140 mm Hg systolic or 90 mm Hg diastolic) or when hypertension is confirmed by home monitoring.

In ambulatory monitoring, an inflatable cuff is worn around the arm and connected to a blood pressure monitor about the size of a Walkman. The monitor is placed in a pouch that is worn at the waist in a holster. At predetermined times—typically every 15 to 30 minutes during the day and every 30 to 60 minutes during the night—the cuff inflates automatically and takes blood pressure readings that are stored in the monitor and later interpreted by a doctor.

While wearing the monitor, people are asked to keep a diary of what time they awoke and went to sleep, when and what they ate, any emotions they experienced, any medications they took, and any physical activity they engaged in. This information may be helpful in explaining fluctuations in blood pressure.

The monitor is lightweight and quiet, and most people are able to sleep and carry out their normal activities while wearing it. Rarely, people may experience minor bruising, swelling, or rash. Medicare covers ambulatory blood pressure monitoring for people with suspected white coat hypertension; most private insurance companies, however, do not cover ambulatory monitoring.

Medical Evaluation of Blood Pressure

Proper diagnosis of hypertension requires a thorough medical history, a physical examination, and laboratory tests. Blood pressure levels determined by a doctor to be lower than 120 mm Hg systolic and 80 mm Hg diastolic should be rechecked within two years. Pressures between 120 and 139 mm Hg systolic or 80 and 89 mm Hg diastolic should be rechecked within one year.

When blood pressure levels are consistently 140/90 mm Hg or above, the next step is to determine whether the hypertension is primary or secondary. Although secondary hypertension is uncommon, secondary causes of high blood pressure should always be considered, since they are correctable in many cases and their identification may spare the patient a lifetime of antihypertensive medication.

Precise diagnosis of a secondary cause usually requires special laboratory tests and procedures. Because these tests are expensive and inconvenient, they are not performed in everyone. Instead, they are done only when a thorough medical history and physical examination—or the results of routine laboratory tests—raise a strong suspicion for a secondary cause of hypertension. The chance that an underlying disorder is responsible for hypertension is particularly likely when lifestyle modifications and a combination of three antihypertensive medications cannot control blood pressure; blood pressure increases unexpectedly in an individual whose blood pressure was previously well controlled; a hypertensive emergency occurs (see pages 7–8); blood pressure increases to greater than 180/110 mm Hg in an individual who previously had normal blood pressure; blood potassium levels drop for no particular reason; or an individual experiences headache, perspiration, and palpitations suggestive of pheochromocytoma (see page 5).

NEW RESEARCH

24-Hour Blood Pressure Monitoring Predicts Strokes, Heart Attacks

For people receiving drug treatment for hypertension, 24-hour ambulatory blood pressure monitoring can help predict who will experience a stroke or heart attack, regardless of their blood pressure readings in the doctor's office, according to researchers.

People with 24-hour ambulatory systolic blood pressures averaging 135 mm Hg or higher were 74% more likely to experience a stroke or heart attack over a five-year period than those with lower 24-hour systolic blood pressures. This result was independent of office blood pressure readings and other traditional risk factors for cardiovascular disease. Ambulatory diastolic blood pressure was also an independent risk factor for stroke or heart attack, but the association was not as strong as it was with systolic blood pressure.

Further research is needed to determine whether 24-hour ambulatory blood pressure monitoring should become part of the standard care for hypertensive patients receiving medication for their condition.

In the study, 1,963 people (average age 56) who were being treated with antihypertensive medication wore blood pressure monitors that took readings every 30 to 60 minutes over a 24-hour period. The participants engaged in their usual activities while wearing the monitors.

THE NEW ENGLAND JOURNAL OF MEDICINE
Volume 348, page 2407
June 12, 2003

Electronic Home Blood Pressure Monitors: How Do They Compare?

When shopping for a home blood pressure monitor, consider whether the monitor is convenient to use, whether the results are consistent, and how much the monitor costs. Also, take time to make sure the cuff fits properly and you are comfortable with how to operate the monitor. In general, arm monitors are recommended over wrist monitors. Some of the less expensive monitors perform better than the more expensive ones.

In 2003, *Consumer Reports* rated 16 top-selling electronic monitors in terms of their consistency and convenience. Nearly all the monitors were found to be highly accurate, so accuracy was not rated. Fingertip models were not included because they are known to be unreliable. The results of the survey are shown below; the models with the highest overall ratings are listed first.

Model	Type	Consistency	Convenience	Overall Rating & Comments	Cost
Omron Automatic BPM with Intellisense HEM-711AC	Arm Automatic	Excellent	Good	**Excellent.** Maker says can be used in people with irregular heartbeat. Has AC adapter.	$80
Omron Automatic BPM HEM-712C or HEM-712CLC	Arm Automatic	Excellent	Fair	**Excellent.** No memory or carrying case.	$70
ReliOn (Wal-Mart) Automatic BPM HEM-741CREL	Arm Automatic	Excellent	Good	**Excellent.** Shorter test time than most. Has AC adapter. No carrying case.	$50
Lifesource One Step Auto-Inflation BPM UA-767V or UA-767VL	Arm Automatic	Excellent	Fair	**Excellent.** Longer test time than most. Single-button operation. Distracting beeps as cuff deflates. Maximum pressure set manually. No memory or carrying case.	$70
Mark of Fitness Auto-Inflate BPM with IQ System MF43	Arm Automatic	Very good	Good	**Very good.** Longer test time than most. Single-button operation. Maker says can be used in people with irregular heartbeat.	$45
Lumiscope Automatic Inflation BPM 1085M or MC	Arm Automatic	Very good	Fair	**Very good.** Distracting beeps as cuff deflates. Maximum pressure set manually. No memory.	$70
Lifesource Quick Response BPM with Easycuff UA-787V	Arm Automatic	Very good	Excellent	**Very good.** Single-button operation. Regular-size cuff easier to use and has wider normal size range than most. Maker says can be used in people with irregular heartbeat.	$85

A careful medical history, physical examination, and routine laboratory tests are also needed to determine whether hypertension has caused tissue or organ damage, to detect lifestyle habits that may be contributing to hypertension, and to identify the presence of additional risk factors for cardiovascular disease.

(Continued)

Model name	Type	Consistency	Convenience	Overall Rating & Comments	Cost
Lumiscope Semi-Automatic BPM 1060	Arm Manual	Very good	Poor	**Very good.** Distracting beeps as cuff deflates. No memory or carrying case. Uses a 9-volt battery.	$35
Lifesource Manual Inflation BPM UA-702V or UA-702VL	Arm Manual	Very good	Poor	**Very good.** Distracting beeps as cuff deflates. No memory or carrying case.	$50
Omron Wrist BPM with APS HEM-637	Wrist Automatic	Very good	Excellent	**Very good.** Less accurate than most. Reads while inflating, so lower cuff pressure. Single-button operation. Cuff easier to use than most. Has correct-position sensor and can graph results.	$125
Healthometer Automatic Digital BPM 7631	Arm Automatic	Good	Good	**Very good.** Shorter test time than most. Reads while inflating, so lower cuff pressure. Single-button operation. No large cuff available at press time. Cuff hard to unfasten.	$85
Lumiscope Smartinflate Blood Pressure & Pulse Monitor 1095	Arm Automatic	Good	Very good	**Very good.** Shorter test time than most. Reads while inflating, so lower cuff pressure. Single-button operation. Monitor attaches conveniently to cuff.	$90
Lifesource Wrist Ultra Compact BPM UB-401	Wrist Automatic	Fair	Good	**Good.** Longer test time than most. Single-button operation. Cuff easier to use than most.	$110
Mark of Fitness Wrist-watch Style BPM MF-75	Wrist Automatic	Fair	Excellent	**Good.** Shorter test time than most. Single-button operation. Cuff easier to use than most. Maker says can be used in people with irregular heartbeat.	$70
Omron Portable Wrist BPM HEM-629	Wrist Automatic	Fair	Very good	**Fair.** Less accurate than most. Shorter test time and cuff easier to use than most.	$75
Lumiscope Fuzzy Logic Automatic Inflation BPM 1091	Wrist Automatic	Fair	Good	**Fair.** Considerably less accurate than most. Longer test time and cuff easier to use than most.	$90

Source: *Consumer Reports*, June 2003.

TREATMENT OF HYPERTENSION

Treatment of primary hypertension involves both lifestyle modifications and antihypertensive medications. The goal of treatment is to lower blood pressure and reduce the risk of complications from hypertension, such as strokes, heart attacks, and kidney disease. Most people with hypertension should aim to lower their blood pressure to less than 140/90 mm Hg. Those with diabetes or kidney disease have an even lower blood pressure goal—less than 130/80 mm Hg.

The same blood pressure goals apply to people with secondary hypertension. In these individuals, however, doctors often try to treat the underlying disorder, especially if blood pressure is difficult to control with lifestyle modifications and medications.

People experiencing a hypertensive emergency (see pages 7–8) must seek immediate medical attention and have their blood pressure lowered with intravenous antihypertensive medication in the hospital. Blood pressure is lowered gradually to avoid precipitous drops in pressure that could lead to a stroke.

Lifestyle Modifications

Lifestyle modifications are essential for both the prevention and treatment of hypertension. Lifestyle modifications proven to lower blood pressure include weight loss in people who are overweight or obese, the Dietary Approaches to Stop Hypertension (DASH) diet, reduced sodium intake, increased potassium intake, regular physical activity, and moderation in alcohol consumption.

These lifestyle modifications not only help lower blood pressure, but also improve the effectiveness of antihypertensive medication and lower the risk of cardiovascular disease. Studies show that the effects of these lifestyle changes are additive, and people who adopt more of them reap the most benefits. In a recent study led by Lawrence Appel, M.D., one of the authors of this White Paper, people with prehypertension or mild hypertension who lost weight, followed the DASH diet, restricted sodium and alcohol intake, and exercised regularly reduced their systolic blood pressure by an extra 4 mm Hg, compared with people who only received advice on these lifestyle modifications (see the sidebar at right).

Weight loss. All people—whether or not they have hypertension—should aim for a body mass index (BMI) between 18.5 and 24.9. People with a BMI of 25 or more are considered overweight. BMI is a measure of weight in relation to height; it can be determined by multiplying weight in pounds by 704 and dividing the result by the square of height in inches. The best way to lose weight is to reduce the number of calories eaten per day while increasing physical activity. Studies show that a 22-lb. weight loss can lower systolic blood pressure by up to 20 mm Hg.

DASH diet. The DASH diet is an eating plan that is rich in

NEW RESEARCH

Combining Lifestyle Modifications Best for Blood Pressure Lowering

Combining as many lifestyle modifications as possible (preferably all of them) is the most effective way to lower blood pressure, according to a new study. This is the first demonstration that combining lifestyle measures can have additive effects on blood pressure.

The study randomly assigned 810 adults, average age 50, who had above-normal blood pressure (120 to 159 mm Hg systolic and 80 to 95 mm Hg diastolic) and were not taking antihypertensive medication to one of three groups. The first group received only advice about lowering blood pressure. The second group adopted numerous lifestyle changes: losing weight if overweight, reducing sodium intake, increasing physical activity, and limiting alcohol. The third group made the same lifestyle changes as the second group but also followed the Dietary Approaches to Stop Hypertension (DASH) diet.

After six months, significantly more people in the lifestyle-plus-DASH group and the lifestyle-only group had normal blood pressure (<120/80 mm Hg) than in the advice-only group (35% and 30% vs. 19%). The results were not statistically different between the lifestyle-plus-DASH group and the lifestyle-only group.

JOURNAL OF THE AMERICAN MEDICAL ASSOCIATION
Volume 289, page 2083
April 23/30, 2003

fruits, vegetables, and low-fat dairy products and low in saturated fat, cholesterol, and total fat. The diet also includes whole-grain products, fish, poultry, and nuts but keeps red meat, sweets, and sugar-containing beverages to a minimum. Two major trials have evaluated the DASH diet.

In the first trial, people who followed the DASH diet for eight weeks reduced their blood pressure by an average of 6/3 mm Hg, compared with people who ate a typical American diet (low in fruits and vegetables and high in fat). The benefits of the DASH diet were most pronounced in people with hypertension. In these individuals, the DASH diet lowered systolic pressure by 11 mm Hg, which is similar to the level of blood pressure reduction typically achieved with a single antihypertensive drug.

In the second trial, people who combined the DASH diet with a low sodium intake (1,500 mg per day) for four weeks had an average blood pressure reduction of 9/5 mm Hg, compared with people who followed a typical American diet with a high sodium intake. As in the first study, the benefits were greater in people with hypertension—their systolic blood pressure dropped by an average of 12 mm Hg.

Sodium restriction. Research indicates that, on average, blood pressure levels rise with higher intakes of sodium, although the effects of sodium on blood pressure are often not apparent in people with hypertension or diabetes or in blacks or older individuals. In general, experts recommend that people consume no more than 2,400 mg of sodium daily. Since sodium is ubiquitous in the typical American diet, reducing sodium intake may require some effort. For starters, stop adding salt at the table and while cooking. Instead, try seasoning foods with salt-free spices or herbs. Since many processed and frozen foods are high in sodium, start reading labels and choose foods that contain less than 140 mg of sodium per serving. Studies show that limiting sodium may lower systolic blood pressure by 2 to 8 mm Hg.

Potassium intake. Potassium is a mineral found in fruits and vegetables. Increased intake of potassium has been shown to reduce blood pressure, as well as to reduce the rise in blood pressure that occurs with excessive salt consumption.

Physical activity. Exercise is also important in the prevention and treatment of hypertension. Experts recommend engaging in moderate physical activity (for example, walking, bicycling, swimming, or jogging) for at least 30 minutes on most days of the week. In a recent meta-analysis of more than 50 randomized, controlled

NEW RESEARCH

DASH Diet Helps Improve Sodium Excretion

The Dietary Approaches to Stop Hypertension (DASH) diet lowers elevated blood pressure, but its mechanism of action has been unclear. A new study shows that the DASH diet works like a diuretic drug, improving the excretion of sodium in the urine.

Researchers randomized 375 people with prehypertension or hypertension to follow either the DASH diet (which is rich in fruits, vegetables, and low-fat dairy foods) or a typical American diet for three 30-day periods. For each period, the sodium level of the diet varied, so that each participant ate a low, moderate, and high-sodium diet in random order.

People following the DASH diet excreted more salt in their urine and lowered their blood pressure more than those receiving the typical diet. The DASH diet was more effective in people with higher sodium intakes (indicating that its main blood pressure-lowering effect is through sodium excretion). Also, the diet was more effective in those with hypertension, in blacks, and in people age 45 and older.

The researchers hypothesize that minerals such as potassium and calcium, which are abundant in the DASH diet, may contribute to its ability to eliminate sodium from the body.

HYPERTENSION
Volume 42, page 8
July 2003

trials, regular physical activity reduced blood pressure by an average of 4/3 mm Hg. For more information on exercise and blood pressure, see the feature on the opposite page. Always talk to your doctor before beginning an exercise program.

Alcohol restriction. Moderate alcohol consumption—one or two drinks a day for most men and one drink a day for women and lighter-weight men—may lower systolic blood pressure by 2 to 4 mm Hg. One drink is equivalent to 12 oz. of beer, 5 oz. of wine, or 1½ oz. of 80-proof spirits. Nondrinkers should not begin drinking to reduce their blood pressure.

Medication

When lifestyle modifications are insufficient to lower blood pressure to goal levels, doctors add antihypertensive medications to the treatment regimen. There are 10 classes of antihypertensive drugs, and each lowers blood pressure in a different way. The best blood-pressure lowering medication or medications for a particular person depends on how severe the hypertension is and whether other health problems are present.

For people with stage 1 hypertension (140 to 159 mm Hg systolic or 90 to 99 mm Hg diastolic) who have no other health problems, a thiazide diuretic is most often prescribed along with lifestyle modifications. In the case of healthy people with stage 2 hypertension (160 mm Hg or higher systolic or 100 mm Hg or higher diastolic), a combination of two drugs is typically prescribed in addition to lifestyle modifications. The drug combination usually consists of a thiazide diuretic and an ACE inhibitor, angiotensin II receptor blocker, beta-blocker, or calcium channel blocker.

Many people with hypertension have other health conditions, and these individuals may require different or additional antihypertensive medications to control their blood pressure and manage their other health problem. For example, people with angina are usually prescribed a beta-blocker or calcium channel blocker to help relieve symptoms. People who have suffered a heart attack typically take an ACE inhibitor, beta-blocker, and aldosterone blocker to prevent another heart attack. In people with severe heart failure, a combination of an ACE inhibitor, beta-blocker, angiotensin II receptor blocker, aldosterone blocker, and loop diuretic is recommended. For people who have had a stroke, taking a thiazide diuretic and an ACE inhibitor can reduce the risk of another stroke.

In people with diabetes, at least two antihypertensive medications are usually required to reach the blood pressure goal of

How Exercise Helps Control Hypertension

Increasing your level of physical activity is a great way to get your blood pressure under control.

Exercise is an important part of the prevention and treatment of hypertension. In combination with other lifestyle measures, such as weight loss and improved diet, regular exercise can help control blood pressure, even in people with normal blood pressure levels and in those taking antihypertensive medication.

People who are physically fit are less likely to develop high blood pressure, and exercise may stop people with prehypertension from developing full-blown hypertension. In people with mild to moderate hypertension, studies have demonstrated that regular aerobic activity can decrease blood pressure by up to 10/8 mm Hg. In some people with hypertension, beginning a regular exercise program can allow their doctors to reduce the dosage of their antihypertensive medication or even eliminate the need for medication altogether.

The Evidence

A 2002 meta-analysis from the *Annals of Internal Medicine* combined the results of 54 randomized, controlled trials that looked at the effect of aerobic exercise on blood pressure in 2,419 people. Most of the studies showed a reduction in blood pressure with regular exercise—an average decrease of 4/3 mm Hg.

This reduction was greater in studies that lasted for fewer than six months, probably because people adhere to exercise regimens better in the short term. Exercise lowered blood pressure whether people had normal or high blood pressure and whether they had a normal body weight or were overweight. Research has also demonstrated that aerobic exercise can lower blood pressure in both older and younger people, and in both men and women.

One study found that half of people taking antihypertensive drugs no longer needed the medication if they jogged two miles a day. Other research shows that regular exercise can lower blood pressure as much as beta-blockers or calcium channel blockers in people with mild to moderate hypertension.

Even modest decreases in blood pressure can reduce the risk of death from all causes, including strokes and coronary heart disease—two potential complications of hypertension. For example, a decrease in blood pressure of 5/5 mm Hg through exercise can lower the risk of a heart attack by 15%.

Exactly how exercise helps to lower blood pressure is unknown. Because exercise reduces blood pressure even in people who do not lose weight, weight reduction is not the only factor involved. Researchers have proposed that exercise may lessen insulin resistance and lower elevated insulin levels, which may in turn affect blood pressure.

Exercise: Types and Intensity

So, which exercises help to lower blood pressure? Studies show that resistance exercises—weight lifting and the use of resistance equipment (like Nautilus machines and resistance bands)—are not an effective way to decrease blood pressure. In fact, in people with hypertension, very high-resistance activities can cause blood pressure to rise, sometimes to dangerous levels.

Nonetheless, experts still recommend the use of resistance exercises as part of an overall exercise plan because these exercises improve strength, balance, and bone mass. But older people and those with hypertension need to take special precautions. For example, they should use light weights (no more than 10 lbs.) and do more repetitions. They may also need to avoid activities that involve heavy lifting, such as shoveling snow.

Aerobic exercises—such as walking, bicycling, swimming, jogging, and dancing—can help lower blood pressure when done for 30 to 60 minutes at least three days a week. If you are unable to exercise for 30 minutes at a time, try breaking up the exercise into sessions of 5 to 10 minutes. Initially, these activities need not be formal exercises but can be everyday activities that you incorporate into your daily routine. For example, try parking your car further away from the store or mall to increase the amount of time you spend walking. When possible, take the stairs instead of an elevator.

Before beginning an exercise program, you need to know what intensity of exercise is beneficial and safe for your age and health status. So, first check with your doctor to determine if you need to take any special precautions.

To reduce blood pressure, the exercise intensity that most people need to reach is 50% to 80% of their maximum heart rate. To determine these numbers, subtract your age from 220; then multiply the result by 0.5 and 0.8, respectively. The resulting numbers are the range of heartbeats per minute that your heart rate should fall into during exercise. Essentially, exercise should cause you to sweat but should not be so intense that you cannot hold a conversation during the activity. You should always warm up and cool down before and after exercising with activities like light walking and stretching.

If you are just getting started, remember that even small increases in physical activity have a beneficial effect not only on your blood pressure but on many other aspects of your health as well.

130/80 mm Hg. The best antihypertensive medications for people with diabetes are those that also lower the risk of diabetes complications. For example, thiazide diuretics, beta-blockers, ACE inhibitors, angiotensin II receptor blockers, and calcium channel blockers reduce the risk of strokes and heart attacks in people with diabetes. In addition, ACE inhibitors and angiotensin II receptor blockers slow the progression of diabetic kidney disease.

People with kidney disease also have a blood pressure goal of 130/80 mm Hg, and they usually need three or more antihypertensive drugs to lower their blood pressure to this level. In these individuals, ACE inhibitors and angiotensin II receptor blockers are most effective in lowering blood pressure and slowing the progression of kidney disease. Because of reduced kidney function, loop diuretics rather than thiazide diuretics are commonly used.

The ten classes of antihypertensive medications are described below and in the chart on pages 26–29.

Diuretics. Often referred to as fluid or water pills, diuretics help reduce blood pressure by increasing the kidneys' excretion of sodium into the urine. These drugs also lower blood pressure by promoting the dilation of small blood vessels. There are three types of diuretics—thiazide diuretics, loop diuretics, and potassium-sparing diuretics. Each type of diuretic acts on a different site in the kidney.

Thiazide diuretics are the most commonly used diuretic. These drugs are inexpensive and need to be taken only once a day. In addition, they are at least as effective—if not more effective—than other classes of antihypertensive drugs at lowering blood pressure and reducing the risk of cardiovascular disease such as strokes and heart attacks. Loop diuretics are often used in people who also have heart failure or kidney disease. Potassium-sparing diuretics are used in combination with another type of diuretic, when that diuretic results in excessive loss of potassium.

Many of the benefits of thiazide diuretics were demonstrated in a recent study called ALLHAT—the Antihypertensive and Lipid-Lowering Treatment to Prevent Heart Attack Trial—published in December 2002 in the *Journal of the American Medical Association.* The study looked at more than 42,000 people with hypertension who were age 55 and older and had at least one risk factor for heart disease. The participants were randomly assigned to receive either a thiazide diuretic (chlorthalidone), an ACE inhibitor (lisinopril), a calcium channel blocker (amlodipine), or an alpha-blocker (doxazosin). The researchers followed the participants for an average of five years.

The results clearly showed that the diuretic was superior to the ACE inhibitor and calcium channel blocker in terms of lowering blood pressure and preventing certain cardiovascular events. (The alpha-blocker portion of the study was stopped early because participants on this medication had a 25% increase in cardiovascular events relative to the diuretic.) People taking the diuretic had systolic blood pressures about 2 mm Hg lower than the group taking the ACE inhibitor and 1 mm Hg lower than the calcium channel blocker group. In addition, people on the diuretic had a lower risk of heart failure compared with people taking the calcium channel blocker and a lower risk of stroke, heart failure, and angina than people treated with the ACE inhibitor.

Side effects of diuretics include weakness; fatigue; malaise; sexual dysfunction; increased blood levels of glucose, triglycerides, calcium, and uric acid; and reduced blood sodium and HDL cholesterol levels. Thiazide and loop diuretics can also cause loss of potassium, which can lead to serious cardiac risks. Low doses of thiazide diuretics are well tolerated, however.

Beta-blockers. These drugs block the actions of epinephrine and lower blood pressure by slowing heart rate and reducing cardiac output (the amount of blood pumped by the heart). They offer the additional benefit of reducing the heart's consumption of oxygen, which can help control angina.

Side effects of beta-blockers include the following: wheezing in people who are sensitive to various allergens and irritants or who have preexisting lung disease; fatigue; drowsiness; malaise; depression; erectile dysfunction or decreased libido; increased blood triglyceride levels; and decreased HDL cholesterol levels. Because beta-blockers blunt the response to epinephrine, these drugs may cause problems if hypoglycemia (low blood sugar) develops in people taking insulin or certain oral drugs to control their diabetes. (Epinephrine release during hypoglycemia triggers symptoms that alert people that their blood sugar is too low and that they need to take actions to increase their blood sugar.)

Beta-blockers may become less effective over time. This happens when the body compensates for the drop in blood pressure by increasing the retention of water and salt, which causes blood pressure to rise again. Combining a beta-blocker with a diuretic may reduce this effect.

Calcium channel blockers. These drugs lower blood pressure by dilating arteries and, depending on the type, by decreasing cardiac output. Like beta-blockers, calcium channel blockers help alleviate

Antihypertensive Drugs 2004

Drug Type	Generic Name	Brand Name	Usual Daily Dosage*	Wholesale Cost (Generic Cost)†
Diuretics	*Thiazide diuretics:*			
	chlorothiazide	Diuril	125 to 500 mg	250 mg: $17 ($12)
	chlorthalidone	Thalitone	12.5 to 25 mg	15 mg: $97 (25 mg: $14)
	hydrochlorothiazide	HydroDIURIL	12.5 to 50 mg	25 mg: $17 ($7)
		Microzide	12.5 to 50 mg	12.5 mg: $60
	indapamide	Lozol	1.25 to 2.5 mg	2.5 mg: $119 ($79)
	metolazone	Mykrox	0.5 to 1 mg	0.5 mg: $124
		Zaroxolyn	2.5 to 5 mg	5 mg: $118
	polythiazide	Renese	2 to 4 mg	2 mg: $69
	Loop diuretics:			
	bumetanide	Bumex	0.5 to 2 mg	0.5 mg: $40 ($30)
	furosemide	Lasix	20 to 80 mg	40 mg: $34 ($16)
	torsemide	Demadex	2.5 to 10 mg	5 mg: $75
	Potassium-sparing diuretics:			
	amiloride	Midamor	5 to10 mg	5 mg: $58 ($48)
	spironolactone	Aldactone	25 to 50 mg	50 mg: $114 ($82)
	triamterene	Dyrenium	50 to 100 mg	50 mg: $95
Beta-blockers	acebutolol	Sectral	200 to 800 mg	200 mg: $210 ($104)
	atenolol	Tenormin	25 to 100 mg	50 mg: $133 ($78)
	betaxolol	Kerlone	5 to 20 mg	10 mg: $106 ($95)
	bisoprolol	Zebeta	2.5 to 10 mg	5 mg: $148 ($121)
	carvedilol‡	Coreg	12.5 to 50 mg	12.5 mg: $173
	labetalol‡	Normodyne	200 to 800 mg	100 mg: $62 ($48)
		Trandate	200 to 800 mg	200 mg: $96
	metoprolol	Lopressor	50 to 100 mg	100 mg: $137 ($76)
	metoprolol, extended release	Toprol XL	50 to 100 mg	100 mg: $114
	nadolol	Corgard	40 to 120 mg	80 mg: $263 ($140)
	penbutolol	Levatol	10 to 40 mg	20 mg: $166
	pindolol	—	10 to 40 mg	(10 mg: $96)
	propranolol	Inderal	40 to 160 mg	80 mg: $130 ($67)
	propranolol, long acting	Inderal LA	60 to 180 mg	80 mg: $149
	timolol	Blocadren	20 to 40 mg	10 mg: $66 ($34)
Calcium channel blockers	amlodipine	Norvasc	2.5 to 10 mg	5 mg: $150
	diltiazem, extended release	Cardizem CD	180 to 420 mg	120 mg: $144 ($126)
		Cardizem LA	120 to 540 mg	120 mg: $130
		Dilacor XR	180 to 420 mg	120 mg: $146 ($126)
		Tiazac	180 to 420 mg	120 mg: $110 ($126)
	felodipine	Plendil	2.5 to 20 mg	5 mg: $121
	isradipine	DynaCirc CR	2.5 to 10 mg	5 mg: $167
	nicardipine, sustained release	Cardene SR	60 to 120 mg	30 mg: $89 ($64)
	nifedipine, long acting	Adalat CC	30 to 90 mg	60 mg: $266
		Procardia XL	30 to 90 mg	30 mg: $157 ($116)
	nisoldipine	Sular	10 to 40 mg	30 mg: $120
	verapamil, immediate release	Calan	80 to 320 mg	120 mg: $99 ($43)
		Isoptin	80 to 320 mg	120 mg: $136 ($43)
	verapamil, long acting	Calan SR	120 to 480 mg	120 mg: $199 ($103)
		Isoptin SR	120 to 480 mg	120 mg: $136 ($103)
	verapamil, controlled onset, extended release	Covera-HS	120 to 480 mg	180 mg: $155 ($132)
		Verelan PM	120 to 480 mg	100 mg: $149 ($132)

Advantages	Disadvantages
Thiazide diuretics are the first drug prescribed for most people with hypertension. These drugs can be used alone or in combination with other antihypertensive drugs, such as ACE inhibitors, angiotensin II receptor blockers, beta-blockers, and calcium channel blockers. Thiazide diuretics may make other antihypertensive drugs more effective by reversing the fluid retention that some of them cause. These drugs are also useful for people with heart failure, since they help to eliminate excess fluid from the body. The thiazide diuretic metolazone is helpful for people with impaired kidney function who do not respond to other thiazides. Loop diuretics sometimes are used for people who are not helped by thiazide diuretics, especially those with impaired kidney function. Potassium-sparing diuretics can be taken alone but generally are used in conjunction with another type of diuretic to counteract excessive potassium loss.	Thiazide diuretics may cause potassium loss, elevated triglyceride and glucose levels, decreased high density lipoprotein (HDL, or "good") cholesterol levels, gout, weakness, erectile dysfunction, and dizziness on standing. Loop diuretics can cause dehydration, potassium loss, and changes in the acidity of the blood. Potassium-sparing diuretics can raise potassium levels, a particular danger for people who have kidney disease. Potassium-sparing diuretics should be used cautiously (if at all) in combination with ACE inhibitors, which can also raise potassium levels.
These drugs are effective for people with hypertension who also have angina or have had a heart attack, since they can help control chest pain and reduce the risk of a second heart attack and death from any cause.	Side effects include fatigue, drowsiness, vivid dreams, loss of libido, and erectile dysfunction. These drugs may also raise triglyceride levels and lower HDL cholesterol levels. High doses may aggravate heart failure. Beta-blockers should not be taken by people with asthma. These drugs are less effective in blacks and the elderly. Abruptly stopping a beta-blocker can produce serious cardiovascular problems.
Calcium channel blockers help relieve the symptoms of angina. Side effects tend to be mild.	Constipation, swelling of the legs, headaches, and dizziness are possible side effects, but most people experience only mild problems, if any. Some classes of calcium channel blockers may aggravate irregular heart rhythms and heart failure. Studies suggest an increased risk of heart attack in users of short-acting calcium channel blockers, but not in people taking longer-acting calcium channel blockers. However, longer-acting calcium channel blockers are associated with an increased risk of heart failure.

* These dosages represent an average range for the treatment of hypertension. The precise effective dosage varies from patient to patient and depends on many factors. Do not make any changes in your medication without consulting your doctor.

† Average wholesale prices to pharmacists for 100 tablets or capsules of the dosage strength listed. Costs to consumers are higher. If a generic version is available, the price is listed in parentheses. Source: *Red Book, 2003* (Medical Economics Data, publishers).

‡ An alpha-blocker and beta-blocker.

Antihypertensive Drugs 2004 (continued)

Drug Type	Generic Name	Brand Name	Usual Daily Dosage*	Estimated Cost (Generic Cost)†
ACE inhibitors	benazepril	Lotensin	10 to 40 mg	10 mg: $105
	captopril	Capoten	25 to 100 mg	12.5 mg: $119 ($69)
	enalapril	Vasotec	2.5 to 40 mg	10 mg: $125 ($105)
	fosinopril	Monopril	10 to 40 mg	10 mg: $107
	lisinopril	Prinivil	10 to 40 mg	10 mg: $107
		Zestril	10 to 40 mg	10 mg: $115
	moexipril	Univasc	7.5 to 30 mg	7.5 mg: $98
	perindopril	Aceon	4 to 8 mg	8 mg: $186
	quinapril	Accupril	10 to 40 mg	10 mg: $118
	ramipril	Altace	2.5 to 20 mg	10 mg: $169
	trandolapril	Mavik	1 to 4 mg	4 mg: $99
Angiotensin II receptor blockers	candesartan	Atacand	8 to 32 mg	16 mg: $145
	eprosartan	Teveten	400 to 800 mg	400 mg: $103
	irbesartan	Avapro	150 to 300 mg	150 mg: $153
	losartan	Cozaar	25 to 100 mg	25 mg: $159
	olmesartan	Benicar	20 to 40 mg	20 mg: $131
	telmisartan	Micardis	20 to 80 mg	20 mg: $151
	valsartan	Diovan	80 to 320 mg	80 mg: $155
Alpha-blockers	carvedilol‡	Coreg	12.5 to 50 mg	25 mg: $173
	doxazosin	Cardura	1 to 16 mg	2 mg: $115 ($93)
	labetalol‡	Normodyne	400 to 800 mg	100 mg: $62 ($48)
	prazosin	Minipress	2 to 20 mg	2 mg: $73 ($47)
	terazosin	Hytrin	1 to 20 mg	2 mg: $212 ($161)
Central alpha agonists	clonidine	Catapres	0.1 to 0.8 mg	0.2 mg: $133 ($33)
	clonidine patch	Catapres TTS	0.1 to 0.3 mg	12 0.1-mg patches: $154
	guanabenz	—	8 to 32 mg	(4 mg: $71)
	guanfacine	—	0.5 to 2 mg	(1 mg: $87)
	methyldopa	Aldomet	250 to 1,000 mg	250 mg: $46 ($35)
Peripheral-acting adrenergic antagonists	guanadrel	Hylorel	20 to 75 mg	10 mg: $200
	guanethidine	Ismelin	25 to 50 mg	5 mg: $63
Direct vasodilators	hydralazine	Apresoline	25 to 100 mg	50 mg: $65 ($8)
	minoxidil	Loniten	2.5 to 80 mg	10 mg: $192 ($129)
Aldosterone blockers	eplerenone	Inspra	50 to 100 mg	n/a

* These dosages represent an average range for the treatment of hypertension. The precise effective dosage varies from patient to patient and depends on many factors. Do not make any changes in your medication without consulting your doctor.

† Average wholesale prices to pharmacists for 100 tablets or capsules of the dosage strength listed. Costs to consumers are higher. If a generic version is available, the price is listed in parentheses. Source: *Red Book, 2003* (Medical Economics Data, publishers).

‡ An alpha-blocker and beta-blocker.

Advantages	Disadvantages
Cause few side effects. Some individuals report improvements in mood. Kidney damage is slowed in people with diabetes who have mild kidney disease, even if they do not have hypertension. These drugs also slow kidney disease progression in people without diabetes. These drugs reduce the risk of death in people with heart failure and those who have had a heart attack. They also prevent heart failure after a heart attack.	Many individuals develop a dry cough. Skin rash may occur. Sense of taste may be altered. ACE inhibitors must be used with caution by those with severely impaired kidney function. These drugs should not be taken by pregnant women or women in their childbearing years (unless they are using effective contraception).
These drugs are effective and cause few side effects. They need only be taken once a day.	In rare cases, these drugs may cause headache, dizziness, or fatigue. They should not be used by pregnant women or women in their childbearing years (unless they are using effective contraception).
Generally well tolerated. These drugs can reduce the symptoms of benign prostatic hyperplasia in men. Doxazosin and terazosin have the added benefit of raising HDL cholesterol levels.	These drugs may cause light-headedness and even fainting in older people, especially with the first dose. They may lose effectiveness over time. When used alone, doxazosin increases the risk of heart failure and strokes.
Side effects tend to be mild and to diminish with continued use. The clonidine patch requires only once-a-week dosing.	Dizziness (especially in older people), drowsiness, depression, dry mouth, constipation, sleep disturbances, and erectile dysfunction may occur. These drugs should not be stopped abruptly.
These drugs are effective for people with severe hypertension and can be combined with other classes of antihypertensive drugs for maximum benefit. Guanethidine does not cause drowsiness.	These drugs can cause diarrhea, and blood pressure may fall rapidly upon standing or with exercise.
Hydralazine can be very effective for people with severe hypertension. Minoxidil is more potent than hydralazine and is especially useful when severe hypertension is accompanied by kidney dysfunction. Combining these drugs with a beta-blocker and a diuretic greatly reduces side effects.	Hydralazine can cause a lupus-like syndrome at high doses. Minoxidil may cause unwanted hair growth. Heart palpitations and swelling of the feet or lower legs are also common.
May be used alone or in combination with other antihypertensive drugs. Works in a broad range of patients.	High blood potassium levels caused by poor kidney function are a rare but serious side effect. Less serious side effects include dizziness, fatigue, flu-like symptoms, diarrhea, and cough.

symptoms of angina. Possible side effects include headache, dizziness, flushing, leg swelling, constipation, and slow or rapid heart rate with palpitations.

Past research suggested that calcium channel blockers might increase the risk of nonfatal heart attacks and deaths due to coronary heart disease, particularly in people treated with short-acting calcium channel blockers such as nifedipine. But in the recently published ALLHAT study, people taking the calcium channel blocker amlodipine (Norvasc) were no more likely to have a heart attack or die of coronary heart disease over a five-year period than people taking the thiazide diuretic chlorthalidone (Thalitone).

However, in ALLHAT, people treated with a calcium channel blocker were 38% more likely to develop heart failure and 35% more likely to be hospitalized for heart failure, compared with people taking a diuretic. Also, other studies have found that calcium channel blockers may adversely affect kidney function, compared with ACE inhibitors. As a result, calcium channel blockers are not recommended as a first-choice treatment for hypertension and should be used cautiously, if at all, in people with heart failure or kidney disease.

ACE inhibitors. ACE inhibitors decrease blood pressure by reducing the formation of angiotensin II, a potent constrictor of blood vessels. These drugs are well tolerated and have no ill effects on libido or erectile function. A dry cough, however, occurs in about 25% of people using ACE inhibitors, especially women. Uncommon adverse effects of ACE inhibitors are rash and increased blood potassium levels. A study comparing two commonly used ACE inhibitors, captopril (Capoten) and enalapril (Vasotec), found that captopril was associated with fewer side effects that decrease quality of life.

The Heart Outcomes Prevention Evaluation (HOPE) trial found that ACE inhibitors are appropriate for a wide range of people. The trial examined the effects of the ACE inhibitor ramipril (Altace) in more than 9,000 people with coronary heart disease, stroke, peripheral vascular disease, or diabetes and at least one other heart disease risk factor (hypertension, elevated cholesterol levels, or smoking). After five years, 14% of the participants taking ramipril had died or suffered a heart attack or stroke, compared with 18% of the patients taking a placebo. This translates into roughly 150 fewer heart attacks or strokes for every 1,000 people treated with ramipril over a four-year period. The ramipril patients were also about 30% less likely to develop diabetes.

In people with diabetes, ACE inhibitors can delay or prevent the progression of kidney disease. These medications are also beneficial in people without diabetes who have early kidney disease. In addition, a recent study found that ACE inhibitors delayed the progression of kidney disease in blacks with early evidence of kidney damage from hypertension. ACE inhibitors must be used with caution, however, when kidney disease is advanced. Furthermore, these drugs should not be used in women who are pregnant or plan to become pregnant.

Angiotensin II receptor blockers. These drugs work by interfering with the action of angiotensin II, which raises blood pressure by constricting small blood vessels and stimulating the adrenal glands to produce the sodium-retaining hormone aldosterone. The drugs may also halt the overgrowth of smooth muscle cells in blood vessel walls. In addition to their blood pressure-lowering effects, angiotensin II receptor blockers also help slow the progression of kidney disease in people with or without diabetes.

Side effects may include headache, digestive upset, and upper respiratory tract infection, although these effects occurred at about the same frequency in people taking a placebo. People who develop a cough while taking an ACE inhibitor may switch to an angiotensin II receptor blocker to eliminate this side effect. Angiotensin II receptor blockers should not be used by pregnant women or women planning a pregnancy.

Alpha-blockers. These drugs decrease blood pressure by blocking nerve impulses that constrict small arteries, thus lowering resistance to blood flow. Alpha-blockers usually are well tolerated and have beneficial effects on HDL cholesterol levels. They may cause orthostatic hypotension (light-headedness on standing), especially in older patients, as well as weakness, fainting, drowsiness, headaches, and heart palpitations. In addition, they can lose their effectiveness over time when not used in combination with a diuretic.

Alpha-blockers are not recommended as a first-choice therapy for hypertension. According to the results of the ALLHAT study, people taking the alpha-blocker doxazosin (Cardura) had 25% more cardiovascular events and were twice as likely to be hospitalized for heart failure as people treated with a diuretic. Alpha-blockers are also prescribed for the treatment of benign prostatic hyperplasia (noncancerous enlargement of the prostate gland).

Central alpha agonists. Like alpha-blockers, these drugs lower blood pressure by blocking nerve impulses that constrict small arteries. Possible side effects include drowsiness, sleep disturbances, depression, dry mouth, constipation, fatigue, erectile dysfunction,

NEW RESEARCH

Morning Blood Pressure Surge Linked to Risk of Strokes

People whose blood pressure rises sharply in the morning are at increased risk for silent or clinical strokes, new research shows.

The research involved 519 people, average age 72, with hypertension. Investigators used magnetic resonance imaging to detect silent strokes. They also performed 24-hour ambulatory blood pressure monitoring and calculated the morning surge in blood pressure by subtracting the average systolic blood pressure during the hour when blood pressure was lowest during sleep from the average systolic blood pressure during the two hours after awakening.

People whose systolic blood pressure rose 55 mm Hg or more upon awakening were much more likely to have evidence of a prior silent stroke than people whose blood pressure rose less than 55 mm Hg in the morning (57% vs. 33%). Also, those with a morning surge in blood pressure were about twice as likely to have a clinical stroke over the next 3½ years than those with no morning surge (19% vs. 7%).

These results may help explain why cardiovascular events are more likely to occur in the morning. People with a morning surge in blood pressure should be taking long-acting antihypertensive drugs and should avoid heavy physical activity in the morning, according to an accompanying editorial.

CIRCULATION
Volume 107, pages 1347 and 1401
March 18, 2003

and dizziness (especially in older people). These drugs should not be stopped abruptly and therefore should be taken only by individuals who are likely to adhere to their medication regimens. Because of a high frequency of side effects, central alpha agonists usually are used only when other medications are unable to control blood pressure adequately. In addition, central alpha agonists may become less effective over time.

Peripheral-acting adrenergic antagonists. These medications reduce resistance to blood flow in small arteries by inhibiting the release of epinephrine and norepinephrine from nerves. Possible side effects include diarrhea and a profound drop in blood pressure when rising from a seated or reclining position or while exercising. These drugs usually are used in people with severe hypertension.

Direct vasodilators. These drugs act directly on the smooth muscle of small arteries, causing these arteries to widen. They must be used in combination with both a diuretic and a beta-blocker to prevent fluid retention and rapid heartbeat. Excessive hair growth is an adverse side effect of minoxidil (Loniten). However, this discovery led to the development of a topical form of the drug for the treatment of baldness. Direct vasodilators are used only in people with hypertension that is difficult to control.

Aldosterone blockers. Eplerenone (Inspra) is the only drug approved in this class of antihypertensive medications. It works by blocking the activity of the hormone aldosterone. Side effects include dizziness, diarrhea, cough, fatigue, and flu-like symptoms. The drug should not be used by people with high blood potassium levels or those taking potassium supplements or potassium-sparing diuretics. People with diabetes or microalbuminuria (small amounts of protein in the urine) should avoid taking eplerenone as well.

Combination therapy. Most people with hypertension require two or more antihypertensive medications to get their blood pressure under control. Combining medications from different classes often results in greater reductions in blood pressure than using a single drug, because the actions of the drugs may complement each other. For example, diuretics reduce blood pressure by increasing the excretion of sodium and water by the kidneys. But in some people this effect stimulates the release of certain blood pressure-raising hormones to compensate for the drop in blood volume. Adding an ACE inhibitor blocks the actions of these hormones and improves blood pressure control.

Combination therapy can be achieved by taking a separate dose

Coping With the Side Effects of Antihypertensive Drugs

You and your doctor can take steps to minimize the impact of these potential side effects on your daily life.

If you are taking medication to control your blood pressure, you may experience symptoms—some of which may be side effects from the medication. Many medication-related side effects diminish with time, but if they persist or are troublesome, your doctor may be able to minimize them by lowering the dosage, switching you to another drug, or prescribing medication to counteract the side effects. Alternatively, some side effects—particularly the less severe ones—can be managed with lifestyle or self-care measures.

The measures you can take for some common side effects of antihypertensive drugs are described below. Always consult your doctor before taking any over-the-counter remedies or making changes to your diet.

Constipation (calcium channel blockers and central alpha agonists). Eat foods high in fiber (such as fruits, vegetables, whole grains, bran, and legumes) and engage in moderate exercise on most days of the week. If these measures aren't helpful, ask your doctor about laxatives.

Dehydration (loop diuretics). Drink plenty of fluids each day. If you consume beverages containing alcohol or caffeine, do so in moderation.

Dizziness, light-headedness, or fainting (all types of antihypertensive medications but especially alpha-blockers). When standing up from a seated position, rise slowly. When getting up from a recumbent position, sit on the edge of the bed with your feet dangling for one to two minutes; then stand up slowly. Be especially careful about rising slowly when getting up in the middle of the night to use the bathroom. Be careful not to overexert yourself during exercise or in hot weather. Also, try to avoid standing for long periods of time and consuming large amounts of alcohol.

Drowsiness (alpha-blockers, beta-blockers, central alpha agonists, and peripheral-acting adrenergic antagonists). Ask your doctor if you can take your medication once a day 30 minutes before bedtime. If you need to take multiple doses each day, ask if the last dose can be taken close to bedtime. Also, try to avoid other medications that can lead to drowsiness, such as antihistamines, sleeping pills, prescription pain relievers, and muscle relaxants.

Dry mouth (central alpha agonists). Try sucking on sugarless candy, chewing sugarless gum, or melting ice cubes in your mouth. If these measures do not provide relief, ask your doctor about a saliva substitute.

Frequent urination at night (beta-blockers and diuretics). Ask your doctor whether you can take your medication in a single dose in the morning after breakfast. If you require more than one dose daily, ask whether you can take the last dose before 6 P.M.

Headaches (ACE inhibitors, alpha-blockers, angiotensin II receptor blockers, calcium channel blockers, and direct vasodilators). Taking a hot shower or bath, pressing a cold pack to the painful area, regular exercise, and deep breathing may relieve headaches. If these measures aren't helpful ask your doctor to recommend a headache medication.

Increased sensitivity to cold (alpha-blockers, beta-blockers, and direct vasodilators). Dress warmly and be sure to keep your ears, hands, and feet covered in cold weather. Take extra precautions when you anticipate prolonged exposure to cold.

Increased sensitivity to sunlight (beta-blockers, direct vasodilators, and diuretics). Try to avoid direct sunlight, particularly between the hours of 10 A.M. and 3 P.M., when the sun's rays are strongest. Protect yourself from the sun by wearing protective clothing (including a wide-brimmed hat and sunglasses) and using sunblock and lip balm with an SPF of at least 15. Do not use sunlamps or tanning beds or booths.

Potassium loss (loop and thiazide diuretics). Increase your intake of potassium-rich foods such as fruits and vegetables. Alternatively, your doctor may add a potassium supplement or a potassium-sparing diuretic to your treatment regimen.

Tender, swollen, or bleeding gums (calcium channel blockers). Practice good dental hygiene by brushing and flossing teeth and massaging gums daily. Have your teeth cleaned regularly by a dentist.

Upset stomach (angiotensin II receptor blockers, beta-blockers, direct vasodilators, and diuretics). Ask your doctor if you can take your medication with meals or with a glass of milk.

of each drug or using fixed-dose combination drugs (formulations of two different drugs combined in a single pill). Most fixed-dose combinations contain a thiazide diuretic (most often hydrochlorothiazide) and an ACE inhibitor, beta-blocker, angiotensin II receptor blocker, or central alpha agonist. A fixed combination of an

ACE inhibitor and a calcium channel blocker is also available.

Fixed-dose combination drugs are more convenient (fewer pills to take each day) and are less expensive than taking each drug individually. Because the fixed-dose combination tends to contain smaller doses of each drug than if the drugs were taken separately, the risk of side effects may be lower as well. In some cases, one drug in the combination prevents the side effects of the other. For example, ACE inhibitors can reduce the leg swelling that often occurs with calcium channel blockers.

However, fixed-dose combinations reduce dosing flexibility—that is, the dosage of each medication in the combination cannot be varied separately. In addition, no large, long-term studies have proven that fixed-dose combinations offer any benefits over taking the two drugs separately. Therefore, fixed-dose combination drugs are most appropriate for people who have found that the combination of the two drugs effectively controls their blood pressure when taken separately at the same doses as in the combination pill.

The J-curve

A few small observational studies have suggested that people taking antihypertensive medication whose diastolic blood pressure is lowered beyond a certain point have a higher risk of heart attacks than hypertensive patients whose pressure is lowered to a lesser degree. This effect is called the J-curve phenomenon: When the number of deaths from heart attacks in people treated with antihypertensive medications is plotted against diastolic blood pressure on a graph, a line connecting the points shows an increase in deaths at the highest and lowest levels of diastolic pressure (the top of the straight part of the J and the top of the curved part of the J, respectively).

Most experts question whether a J-curve phenomenon exists, particularly in people with hypertension who do not have cardiovascular disease. The Hypertension Optimal Treatment (HOT) study, which involved 18,790 people with hypertension who had diastolic blood pressures between 100 and 105 mm Hg, showed that aggressive reduction of blood pressure to 140/85 mm Hg or lower was associated with a dramatic reduction in the risk of heart attacks. When blood pressure fell even further (for example, to 120/70 mm Hg), there was little additional benefit but also no significant additional risk, thus calling into question the J-curve phenomenon.

Medical Follow-up

People with stage 1 hypertension who are otherwise healthy typically are seen by their doctor once a month until they reach their blood pressure goal. Those with other health problems or stage 2 hypertension need to visit their doctor more frequently—every two to four weeks. At these visits, the doctor may adjust drug doses, add another drug, switch a medication if side effects are troublesome, and inquire about lifestyle modifications.

Once blood pressure is at goal or stabilizes, doctor visits are usually reduced to every three to six months, though people with other health conditions (such as diabetes or heart disease) may need to visit their doctor more often. Levels of blood sodium, potassium, and creatinine should be measured at least once or twice a year to detect any adverse effects from antihypertensive drugs and any deterioration in kidney function.

Only about a third of people with hypertension have reached the blood pressure goal of 140/90 mm Hg. One reason is that some doctors are not treating hypertension aggressively enough; another is that some people are not taking their antihypertensive medications as prescribed or adopting the recommended lifestyle modifications.

Poor compliance with antihypertensive therapy is understandable, considering that many people with hypertension have no or minimal symptoms yet are expected to make lifestyle modifications and take medication that may be costly or cause unpleasant side effects. Nonetheless, compliance is crucial to prevent the complications that may result from high blood pressure. On average, antihypertensive therapy is associated with a 35% to 40% lower risk of a stroke, a 20% to 25% reduced risk of a heart attack, and a 50% decrease in the risk of heart failure.

Stroke

Each year, about 700,000 people in the United States suffer a new or recurrent stroke, and about 167,000 of them die. The number of deaths from stroke rose from 1990 to 2000, but because the population also increased during that time, the number of strokes per 100,000 people fell by about 12%. This fall is probably the result of more aggressive treatment of risk factors for stroke (such as hypertension), earlier diagnosis of stroke, and better medical management of the disease.

NEW RESEARCH

Women Experience Strokes Later But Have More Disability

First strokes tend to occur at an older age and be more disabling in women than in men, according to investigators. These factors may account for the longer hospital stays and more frequent complications experienced by women after a first stroke.

The study analyzed 1,581 people with a first stroke. Women were about six years older than men (75 vs. 69) at the time of the stroke, and the risk factors for stroke were different for men and women. Hypertension and cardioembolic disease (conditions like atrial fibrillation that can cause blood clots to form in and break loose from the heart and travel to the brain) were most predictive of stroke in women, while peripheral vascular disease, smoking, and excessive alcohol intake were more predictive of stroke in men.

In addition, women were more likely than men to suffer from language, vision, and swallowing problems after a stroke. Women were 87% more likely to be disabled and 36% more likely to have in-hospital complications than men, and they had longer hospital stays (15.4 days vs. 13.5 days).

To prevent stroke more effectively, women and their doctors should take steps to control hypertension and to prevent atrial fibrillation with anticoagulant drugs, the authors write.

STROKE
Volume 34, page 1581
July 2003

The news from stroke researchers is encouraging as well. In addition to alteplase (Activase)—the first drug capable of halting a stroke in progress if administered soon enough after stroke onset—other drugs may soon be available for the emergency treatment of a stroke. In addition, researchers are developing new approaches to rehabilitation, which could help people recover more fully and quickly from a stroke. Still, the best weapon against stroke is prevention. More than half of all strokes could be averted if people took the appropriate preventive steps.

THE BRAIN'S BLOOD SUPPLY

Although the brain accounts for only about 2% of the body's weight, it receives some 20% of the oxygenated and nutrient-rich blood pumped from the heart. Two pairs of arteries—the carotid arteries and the vertebral arteries—carry this large volume of blood to the brain.

The left and right carotid arteries receive blood from the heart and transport it up both sides of the front of the neck. As the two carotid arteries approach the top of the neck, each splits into an external carotid artery and an internal carotid artery. The external carotid arteries carry blood to the scalp, face, and neck, while the internal carotid arteries channel blood to the front two thirds of the brain and the eyes.

The left and right vertebral arteries run up the back of the neck, parallel to the spine. At the base of the skull, the two vertebral arteries join to form the basilar artery. Branches from the vertebral and basilar arteries bring blood to the brain stem—the lower portion of the brain near the spine—and to the rear third of the brain.

WHAT IS A STROKE?

A stroke occurs when an artery supplying blood to a portion of the brain becomes blocked or ruptures. As a result, neurons (nerve cells) in the affected area are starved of the oxygen and nutrients they need to function properly.

One reason a stroke is so dangerous is that the brain—unlike muscle or other tissues—has little or no reserve stores of energy. Consequently, when blood flow is interrupted to a part of the brain, some function may be lost in as little as four minutes. And after a few hours of interrupted blood flow, neurons cannot survive. Fortunately, the brain has some natural protection against such interruptions of blood supply—a ring of blood vessels called the circle of Willis at the base of the brain. This structure helps protect neurons by connecting the brain's front and rear blood supplies and providing alternative pathways for blood flow should a major artery become blocked.

Nerve cell damage due to a stroke is usually permanent. But despite the death of neurons, some improvement usually occurs over time as other neurons take over the functions of the neurons that were lost.

TYPES OF STROKE

There are two basic types of stroke: ischemic and hemorrhagic. Even though distinctly different mechanisms are responsible for each, hypertension increases the risk of both. Proper diagnosis of the stroke type is essential for determining the best course of treatment.

Ischemic Stroke

About 88% of all strokes are ischemic, resulting from a blockage in a blood vessel leading to or in the brain. Neurons are damaged not only by the lack of oxygen and nutrients but also by a powerful chain of chemical reactions known as the ischemic (or glutamate) cascade, which leads to a buildup of toxins that further contributes to cell destruction. The degree and duration of an ischemic stroke determine whether the brain suffers temporary impairment, irreversible damage to a few highly vulnerable neurons, or extensive neurological damage.

Cerebral thrombosis. The most common cause of ischemic stroke is cerebral thrombosis. Cerebral thrombosis occurs when a thrombus (blood clot) forms along the wall of one of the major arteries supplying the brain and completely blocks blood flow through the artery. These arteries include the carotid and vertebral arteries, which run along the front and back of the neck, respectively, as well as smaller arteries within the brain itself. Clots are most likely to develop in arteries that are already narrowed by atherosclerotic plaque—the same fatty deposits that cause coronary heart disease. The hard, rough, uneven surfaces of these plaques provide ideal sites for the formation and growth of blood clots, which may eventually completely block the already narrowed artery.

Cerebral embolism. Another possible cause of ischemic stroke is cerebral embolism. It most often occurs when part of a blood clot or a piece of atherosclerotic plaque breaks off and travels through the bloodstream (embolus) until it lodges in an artery supplying the

NEW RESEARCH

Flu Shot Decreases Risk of Stroke, Heart Attack

An annual flu vaccine may reduce the risk of a stroke or heart attack, as well as of dying of any cause, according to a new study.

Researchers studied two groups of people over age 65: 140,055 adults in the 1998 to 1999 flu season and 146,328 in the 1999 to 2000 flu season. In the earlier flu season, 56% of the participants received a flu shot, as did 60% of the participants in the later flu season. Adults who received a flu shot were 20% less likely to be hospitalized for a stroke during both seasons. The flu shot was also associated with a reduced risk during each season of being hospitalized for heart disease by about 19%, being hospitalized for flu or pneumonia by 30%, and dying of any cause by 49%.

It has been theorized that the flu may make strokes and heart attacks more likely by affecting blood clotting or blood vessel dilation, or by causing dehydration. It is also possible that people who get the vaccine tend to engage in other healthy habits that lower their risk.

The flu vaccine was associated with similar benefits for healthy, older adults as well as those with health problems, and the researchers stress the importance of the flu vaccine for all adults over the age of 65. In 2001, only 63% of American adults over age 65 received the flu vaccine.

THE NEW ENGLAND JOURNAL OF MEDICINE
Volume 348, page 1322
April 3, 2003

The Two Major Types of Ischemic Stroke

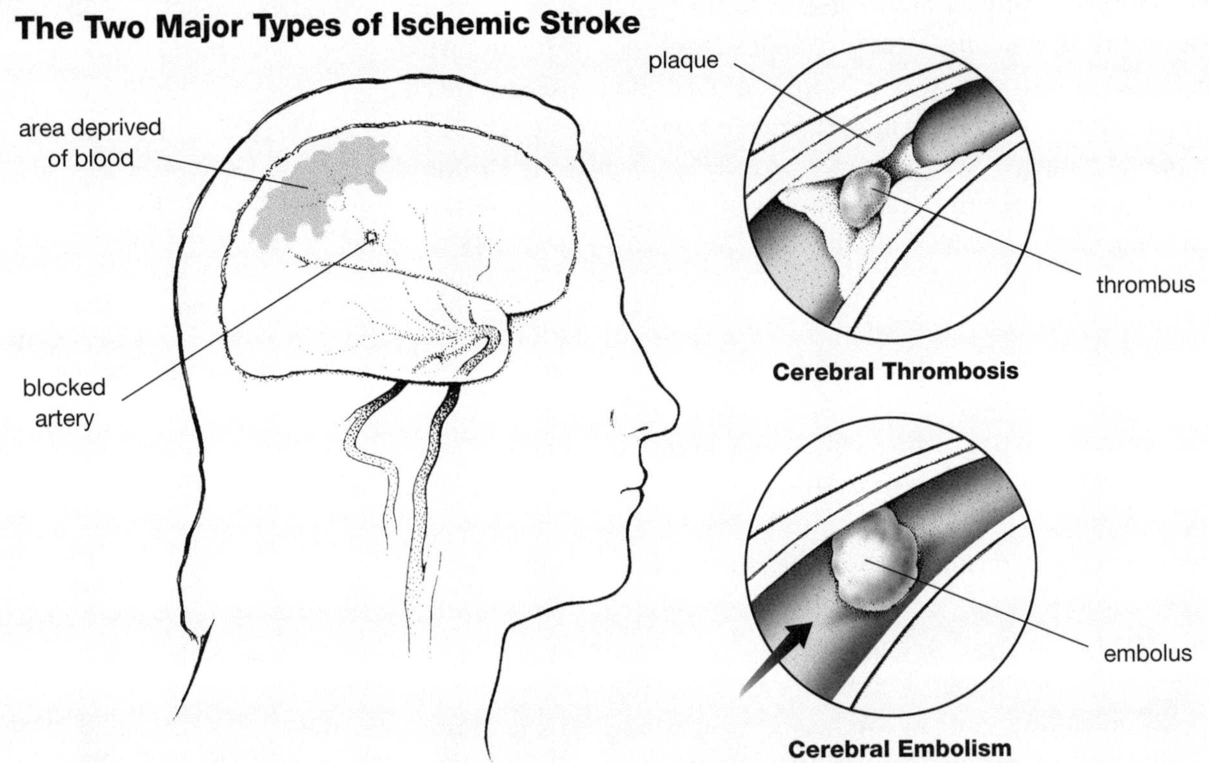

Most strokes are ischemic. They occur when an artery becomes blocked and causes a serious deficit in the blood supply to part of the brain. The most common cause of an ischemic stroke is cerebral thrombosis, in which a blood clot (thrombus) forms in an artery leading to the brain or within the brain itself, usually at a site already narrowed by atherosclerotic plaque. An ischemic stroke may also result when a blood clot or fragment of plaque (embolus) forms in an artery elsewhere in the body and travels through the bloodstream until it becomes wedged in an artery supplying the brain—a condition known as cerebral embolism.

Both types of ischemic stroke can completely cut off blood flow to the region of the brain supplied by the blocked artery. The nerve cells normally nourished by the artery are deprived of the oxygen and nutrients they need to function. If blood flow is not restored quickly, these cells will die, causing permanent impairment in the parts of the body controlled by the affected brain tissue.

brain and blocks blood flow. Most emboli originate in the heart or in large arteries such as the carotid artery. Emboli can also be composed of platelets, an air bubble, or bits of fat released from the marrow of a broken bone.

One of the most common causes of emboli is atrial fibrillation, an abnormal heart rhythm in which the atria (the upper chambers of the heart) quiver chaotically instead of contracting in a rhythmic pattern. The atria may not empty completely of blood; any blood remaining in one place too long tends to stagnate and form blood clots. These blood clots can escape from the heart and travel along the increasingly narrow branches of blood vessels, ultimately lodging in an artery anywhere in the body, but usually in the brain. One third of individuals with untreated atrial fibrillation suffer a stroke during their lifetime.

People with heart muscle damage from a recent heart attack, a poorly functioning heart (for example, due to cardiomyopathy), a diseased heart valve (for example, mitral stenosis), and, possibly, atherosclerotic plaque in the aorta (the main artery emerging from the heart) also are at risk for blood clots that can break off and cause a stroke.

Lacunar strokes. Lacunar strokes are often seen in older people with high blood pressure. They occur when the tiny arterioles (the endmost branches of arteries) that penetrate deep into the brain become completely blocked by small emboli or atherosclerotic plaque. As a result of the blockages, small areas of brain tissue degenerate, leaving behind little cavities called lacunes (lakes). Because the blood vessels involved are so small, symptoms of lacunar strokes are usually mild, and diagnosis may be difficult.

Transient ischemic attacks (TIAs). TIAs are short-lived neurological deficits that result from a temporary blockage of blood flow to the brain. Most episodes subside within 5 to 20 minutes and rarely continue for more than a few hours. Because TIAs do not result in permanent neurological deficits and are almost never painful, people tend to ignore them. But TIAs are an important warning sign of an impending stroke and warrant prompt medical attention. People may have repetitive episodes of TIAs in the days or weeks before a stroke, and one third of those who experience a TIA have a stroke within five years.

Recognition and treatment of the cause of a TIA may help to prevent a stroke and its complications. For example, if carotid stenosis (narrowing of one of the carotid arteries supplying the brain) is detected, a surgical procedure called carotid endarterectomy (see pages 55–58) can be performed.

Hemorrhagic Stroke

Accounting for about 12% of all strokes, hemorrhagic strokes occur when an artery in the brain suddenly bursts and blood leaks out into the surrounding tissue. The bleeding can take place either into the brain itself (intracerebral hemorrhage) or into the space between the brain and the skull (subarachnoid hemorrhage).

Damage occurs in two ways. First, the blood supply is cut off to the parts of the brain beyond the site of the arterial rupture. Second—and posing the greatest danger—the escaped blood forms a mass that exerts excessive pressure on the brain. Blood continues to leak until it clots or until the pressure inside the skull is equal to the blood pressure in the ruptured artery.

Aneurysms—blood-filled pouches that balloon out from weak spots in a blood vessel wall—cause many hemorrhagic strokes. While some aneurysms are congenital (present at birth), they may be exacerbated or even caused by hypertension. Most strokes due to a ruptured aneurysm occur in people between the ages of 40 and 60. Aneurysms are more common in people with polycystic kidney disease (a rare inherited condition in which the kidneys contain multiple cysts) and in those with two or more close relatives with aneurysms. Magnetic resonance angiography (see page 64) can be used to detect large aneurysms.

Brain hemorrhage may also result from a congenital blood vessel defect known as an arteriovenous malformation, which is characterized by a complex, tangled web of arteries and veins. The walls of these abnormal blood vessels tend to be so thin that surges in blood pressure, or simply the wear and tear of normal blood flow, may eventually cause an arteriovenous malformation to rupture and bleed into the brain.

Intracerebral hemorrhage. Intracerebral hemorrhage is characterized by leakage of blood into tissue deep within the brain, usually the cerebrum (the part of the brain that controls higher functions such as speaking and reasoning). Hypertension is the primary cause of intracerebral hemorrhage; other causes include head injury, aneurysm, brain tumor, and illicit drugs such as cocaine and amphetamines. In people over age 80, a common cause of intracerebral hemorrhage is amyloid angiopathy—a weakening of blood vessels by deposits of amyloid, a starch-like substance.

Subarachnoid hemorrhage. Subarachnoid hemorrhage results from bleeding into the space between the brain and the protective arachnoid membrane that lies between the brain and the skull. Most subarachnoid hemorrhages result from a ruptured aneurysm. Head injuries, arteriovenous malformations, and other blood vessel defects also may be responsible. Some 80% of subarachnoid hemorrhages occur in people age 40 to 65; 15%, in those age 20 to 40; and 5%, in those under age 20. Women, especially during pregnancy, are at slightly higher risk for subarachnoid hemorrhage than men.

SYMPTOMS OF STROKE

Like a heart attack, a stroke is an emergency that requires immediate medical attention. Yet, while most people know and can recognize the characteristic symptoms of a heart attack, many are unaware of

The Two Major Types of Hemorrhagic Stroke

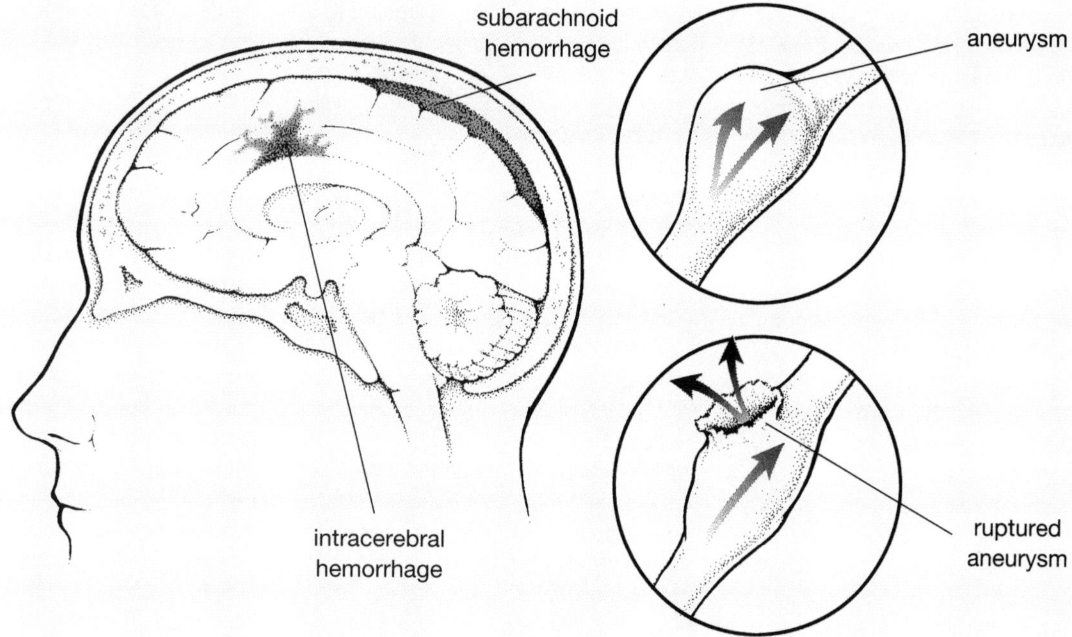

A hemorrhagic stroke occurs when an artery supplying the brain bursts and blood leaks into the surrounding tissue. Depending on the site of the rupture, bleeding may occur within the brain (intracerebral hemorrhage) or between the layers of its protective outer membranes (subarachnoid hemorrhage). Nerve cells in the area are destroyed owing to the disrupted blood supply and also to the pressure from the accumulation of leaking blood. The severity of damage depends on the amount of blood that escapes.

Intracerebral hemorrhages are most often caused by a tear in a small blood vessel in the brain, usually associated with high blood pressure. The subarachnoid type usually occurs at the site of an aneurysm—a bulge that balloons out from a weak spot in an artery wall. Aneurysms may develop in people genetically predisposed to arterial defects, but often hypertension causes them to burst.

the symptoms of a stroke. Moreover, symptoms of a TIA may appear suddenly and then subside just as quickly, creating the false impression that a serious problem does not exist.

The feature on page 42 describes in detail the symptoms of a stroke and the appropriate steps to take if these symptoms occur. Anyone who experiences the sudden onset and persistence of any of the symptoms of stroke must call 911 or go straight to the hospital. Rapid diagnosis and treatment may minimize damage to brain tissue and improve the chance of survival.

EFFECTS OF STROKE

In addition to the initial symptoms, strokes generally produce lasting neurological deficits that may impair a person's senses, motor skills, behavior, language ability, memory, or thought processes. The

If a Stroke Occurs

Like a heart attack, a stroke is an emergency that requires immediate medical attention. Since drug therapy is most likely to be effective within the first three hours of stroke onset, getting to the hospital as soon as symptoms start is essential. Listed below are the symptoms of a stroke, as well as what to do.

Symptoms of Stroke

- Sudden weakness or numbness in the face, arm, or leg on one side of the body.
- Sudden loss, blurring, or dimness of vision.
- Mental confusion, loss of memory, or sudden loss of consciousness.
- Slurred speech, loss of speech, or problems understanding others.
- Sudden, severe headache with no apparent cause.
- Unexplained dizziness, drowsiness, incoordination, or falls.
- Nausea and vomiting, especially when accompanied by any of the above symptoms.

Actions To Take

- Stay calm. Ignore any tendency to downplay a symptom; it's common for people to deny the possibility of something as serious as a stroke. Don't hesitate to take prompt action.
- Call or have someone call an ambulance. (Dial 911 in most parts of the United States.) Be sure to give your name, telephone number, and exact whereabouts.
- While waiting for the ambulance, the person suffering the stroke should be made as comfortable as possible and should not eat or drink anything other than water.
- If an ambulance cannot arrive for an extended period of time, a family member or neighbor should drive the stroke patient to the hospital. Under no circumstances should the person experiencing the stroke symptoms attempt to drive.
- Notify the stroke patient's doctor. He or she can provide the hospital with the patient's medical history, which may be important for determining the best type of treatment.
- At the hospital, be sure to list any medical conditions the stroke patient has (such as high blood pressure), any allergies the patient has (particularly to medication), and any medications the patient is currently taking.

deficits that occur depend on which portions of the brain are damaged by the stroke (as well as on the type and severity of the stroke). Strokes can affect the following areas of the brain: the brain stem, cerebellum, limbic system, and cerebrum.

The Brain Stem, Cerebellum, and Limbic System

At the base of the brain (at the top of the spinal cord) lies the brain stem. The brain stem maintains basic life support functions—breathing, heart rate, blood pressure, and digestion. An extensive stroke affecting the brain stem is usually fatal; when patients do survive, artificial life support is often necessary. Since the brain stem also helps maintain consciousness, a major stroke in this area can result in a coma. A coma also can occur when a stroke in the cerebrum, which surrounds the brain stem, causes swelling that puts pressure on the brain stem.

Above the brain stem is the cerebellum, which controls coordination, balance, and posture. Early symptoms of a stroke in the cerebellum include dizziness, nausea, and vomiting. Later symptoms include clumsiness, shaking, or difficulty controlling certain muscles.

Above the cerebellum is a group of structures known as the limbic system. The limbic system is responsible for the primal urges and powerful emotions that ensure self-preservation: rage, terror, hunger, and sexual desire. Growth and reproductive cycles also are governed by the limbic system. Strokes in this area are rare, but when they do occur, basic drives may be severely limited, or patients may lose their natural inhibitions.

The Cerebrum

Surrounding the brain stem, cerebellum, and limbic system is the cerebrum—the largest portion of the brain and a common site of strokes. Its convoluted outer layer of gray matter, known as the cortex, is the center of conscious thought, perception, voluntary movement, and integration of all sensory input.

The cortex of the cerebrum is divided into two halves, or hemispheres, each responsible for a different set of duties. In most right-handed people, the right hemisphere specializes in spatial relationships, color perception, visual interpretation, and musical aptitude, while the left half of the brain typically oversees analytical tasks (such as mathematical computation and logical reasoning) and linguistic tasks (such as comprehending words and formulating speech). In left-handed people, the hemispheres responsible for these duties are typically reversed. One exception is speech, which usually involves both hemispheres in left-handed people.

Each hemisphere also governs movement and sensory perception on the opposite side of the body. Consequently, a stroke in the left hemisphere can result in paralysis on the right side of the body. Each hemisphere is further subdivided into four distinct sections, known as lobes. The two hemispheres constantly communicate with one another via a thick neural connecting cable known as the corpus callosum.

Frontal lobe. The frontal lobe is situated at the front of the brain, behind the brow. One of the responsibilities of this lobe is motor function—neurons in the motor cortex of the frontal lobe send signals that initiate muscle activity throughout the body. Damage to the motor cortex on one side of the brain can result in weakness or paralysis somewhere on the opposite side of the body. In addition to paralysis of the limbs and torso, muscles on one side of the face or mouth may be affected, altering the person's appearance or ability to speak clearly (a condition called dysarthria). The frontal lobe manages more abstract types of movement as well, including activities that require sequential steps. Consequently, a stroke may make it difficult or impossible to carry out a complex task, such as preparing a meal.

Expressive aphasia—difficulty in speaking, writing, or gesturing—

NEW RESEARCH

Fatal Strokes More Common in Stressed People

People who experience stress frequently and at high intensity are at greater risk for a fatal stroke than people who aren't as stressed, a new study of more than 12,000 adults shows. However, the study's authors are unsure whether stress itself puts people at risk for stroke or whether other factors related to stress are the true causes of the association.

In the Danish study, adults who initially reported a high intensity of stress were nearly two times more likely to have a fatal stroke over the next 13 years than those who reported having no stress. In addition, those who said they had stress at least weekly were 49% more likely to have a fatal stroke during the follow-up period than those who said they never or hardly ever felt stress. No association was found between stress and nonfatal strokes, however.

There are many possible explanations for the relationship between stress and fatal strokes. Stressed people may be more likely to experience more severe strokes or be more vulnerable to complications from stroke. Stress may also contribute to high blood pressure and atherosclerosis—two strong risk factors for stroke. Lastly, stress may cause people to engage in unhealthy behaviors, like smoking or excessive drinking, which can contribute to stroke.

STROKE
Volume 34, page 856
April 2003

can result when a stroke affects the frontal lobe in the dominant hemisphere (for example, the left hemisphere of someone who is right-handed). Insight, initiative, and social inhibitions are governed by the foremost portion of the frontal lobe. A stroke in this area could result in uncharacteristically impulsive or uninhibited behavior. Conversely, profound apathy, lethargy, and a lack of intentional behavior may result—a condition known as abulia.

Parietal lobe. Behind the frontal lobe is the parietal lobe, which is responsible for receiving and interpreting sensory information from all parts of the body. Common problems resulting from a stroke in the parietal lobe are sensory loss, numbness, and vision loss on the side of the body opposite from the brain damage. Damage to the highly specialized sensory cortex in the parietal lobe may result in agnosia, in which the person is unable to interpret incoming visual, auditory, or tactile stimuli, even though the senses of vision, hearing, and touch are mechanically intact and function normally.

Another common consequence of a stroke in the parietal lobe is neglect. People exhibiting neglect typically stop perceiving or acknowledging events, and even sensations, on the side of the body opposite the affected hemisphere.

Temporal lobe. The temporal lobe—situated at ear level, underneath both the parietal and frontal lobes—is dedicated to auditory perception and storage of memories. Strokes in the temporal lobe rarely cause hearing loss; however, they commonly result in language deficits known as aphasia—problems understanding speech, verbalizing thoughts, reading, or writing. Memory loss is also a common consequence of stroke in the temporal lobe. However, memory deficits may be only temporary, since the temporal lobe on the other side of the brain can eventually compensate (unless both sides of the brain have been affected by the stroke).

Occipital lobe. The occipital lobe lies at the rear of the cerebral cortex, in the back of the skull. It is dedicated entirely to the perception and interpretation of visual data delivered from the eyes via the optic nerve. A stroke on the right side of the occipital lobe does not cause blindness in the left eye; instead, it causes hemianopia—blindness in the left field of vision of both eyes. An occipital lobe stroke can also result in loss of the ability to recognize and interpret visual stimuli (for example, faces).

Other Consequences

Besides the deficits described above, a stroke may produce other long-term complications, including impaired concentration, poor judgment, erratic sleep patterns, loss of libido, emotional instability, depression, and seizures. Also, immobility following a stroke may lead to aspiration pneumonia (inhalation of food and other particles into the lungs due to an inability to swallow and cough properly), bedsores, deep vein thrombosis (formation of painful blood clots in the legs), limb contractures (tightening of the muscles in the limbs), incontinence, and urinary tract infection.

RISK FACTORS FOR STROKE

A number of factors contribute to the overall chance of having a stroke. Some of them, such as age or race, obviously cannot be modified. Fortunately, other major risk factors can be significantly reduced through lifestyle measures, medical treatment, or a combination of both. One of these modifiable risk factors is hypertension, which not only accelerates the development of atherosclerosis—the arterial narrowing that accounts for at least two thirds of all ischemic strokes—but is the most important precursor of hemorrhagic stroke.

Risk Factors That Cannot Be Changed

The following important risk factors for stroke cannot be changed. Their presence, however, should alert people to their greater stroke risk and the need to reduce risk factors that they can change.

Age. Between the ages of 55 and 85, the risk of stroke doubles with each successive decade. Only 28% of people who suffer a stroke are younger than age 65.

Gender. Overall, the risk of stroke is approximately 30% higher in men than in women, and this difference is even greater in people younger than age 65. This gender difference is due to many factors, including higher cholesterol levels in men and the protective effect of estrogen in premenopausal women. Men also have a slightly higher risk of dying of stroke than women.

Family history. Stroke risk is greater in people whose close relatives (parents or siblings) have had a stroke.

Race. Blacks have about twice the risk of death and disability from a stroke than whites. Asian-Pacific Islanders and those of Hispanic descent also are at higher risk than whites.

Prior history of stroke. People who have had a stroke are at substantial risk for having another; about 13% have another stroke within a year, and the risk of stroke in each successive year after that is 6%.

NEW RESEARCH

Eating Fruit May Reduce Risk of Ischemic Stroke

Fruits and vegetables may offer some protection against ischemic stroke, according to a new study.

Researchers in Denmark assessed the dietary habits of more than 54,000 men and women, age 50 to 64, between 1993 and 1997. Approximately three years later, 266 participants had experienced an ischemic stroke.

After adjusting for other stroke risk factors such as blood pressure, smoking history, and total calorie intake, people with the highest intake of fruits and vegetables (an average of 22 oz. per day) were 28% less likely to have an ischemic stroke than people with the lowest intake (an average of less than 5 oz. per day). The association was strongest for fruit: People who ate the most fruit were 40% less likely to have an ischemic stroke than people who ate the least.

When the data on individual fruits and vegetables were examined, citrus fruits were associated with the greatest reduction in stroke risk, while mushrooms, onions, garlic, and stalk vegetables (such as leeks and asparagus) were not associated with a reduction in risk. Low potassium intake has been linked with increasing stroke risk; fruits (especially bananas) tend to be high in potassium.

AMERICAN JOURNAL OF CLINICAL NUTRITION
Volume 78, page 57
July 2003

C-Reactive Protein: A New Risk Factor for Stroke

C-reactive protein may be a better predictor of stroke than cholesterol levels. Should you be tested for it?

In the past few decades, physicians have gained considerable knowledge about what causes cardiovascular events like strokes and heart attacks. They have also become increasingly skilled at predicting who will experience these events. Still, some people who have a stroke or heart attack have no known risk factors for the condition. Therefore, researchers are continually searching for additional ways to predict cardiovascular events. One new way may be testing for blood levels of a substance called C-reactive protein (CRP).

CRP, a blood marker for inflammation, is elevated in people who go on to have a stroke or heart attack. At first, researchers thought that CRP might be just a marker for other risk factors—such as smoking, high blood pressure, or high low density lipoprotein (LDL) cholesterol levels—that are known to increase the risk of cardiovascular events. Now researchers believe that increased CRP levels result from inflammation associated with atherosclerosis, and new evidence indicates that CRP may directly contribute to cardiovascular events. A cell study published in *Circulation* in January 2003 showed that elevated CRP levels in the blood may promote clots that can lead to ischemic strokes.

What Is CRP?

CRP is a protein produced by the liver when inflammation occurs in the body. Such inflammation can result from the following:

- atherosclerosis;
- gingivitis;
- rheumatoid arthritis;
- high blood pressure;
- inflammation of the arteries, for example, temporal arteritis;
- obesity;
- metabolic syndrome;
- diabetes;
- smoking; and
- infection (either bacterial or viral).

In fact, some research indicates that a bacterial or viral infection of the arteries may be one of the causes of atherosclerosis.

CRP levels are determined with a blood test. People with CRP levels above 3 mg/L are at increased risk for stroke and other cardiovascular events. Levels between 1 and 3 mg/L confer an average risk for these events, and levels below 1 mg/L are associated with a low risk.

The Evidence

One recent study from Hawaii, published in *Circulation* in April 2003, provides the strongest evidence to date that elevations in CRP levels are associated with an increased risk of ischemic stroke, particularly in those without major risk factors for cardiovascular disease. The investigators compared CRP levels in blood samples taken between 1967 and 1970 from 259 men (age 48 to 69) who had an ischemic stroke in the next 20 years and 1,348 similar men who did not have a stroke during this time. In the entire group, those with the highest CRP levels were almost four times more likely to have a stroke than those with the lowest CRP levels. The association between CRP and ischemic stroke occurred almost exclusively in men who were age 55 or younger, who had never smoked, and who did not have hypertension or diabetes.

A study published in *Circulation* in July 2003 confirmed that CRP is associated with a higher risk of stroke but added that elevated CRP levels appear to be associated with more unstable atherosclerotic plaque than lower CRP levels. Unstable plaque is more likely to rupture and lead to a stroke.

An earlier report, published in *Stroke* in 2002, found that people with elevated CRP levels were twice as likely to experience progression of atherosclerosis in their carotid arteries as people with low CRP. Blood levels of CRP were as effective as blood cholesterol levels, blood pressure, and smoking status at predicting atherosclerosis progression

Another report, published in *The New England Journal of Medicine* in 2002, found that women with low LDL cholesterol but high CRP levels were slightly more likely to have cardiovascular disease than women

Transient ischemic attacks (TIAs). While only about 10% of strokes are preceded by TIAs, these short-lived events are a strong predictor of an eventual full-blown stroke. A stroke is almost 10 times more likely in someone who has experienced a TIA than in someone who has not. Eventually, about 36% of people who have had one or more TIAs will have a stroke. Studies show that between 25% and 50% of TIAs are the result of a blood clot at a site

with low CRP but high LDL cholesterol levels. These data led the study's authors to conclude that CRP "is a stronger predictor of future cardiovascular events than LDL cholesterol."

Should You Be Tested?
The test for CRP is easy to perform (it involves drawing blood from a vein in your arm) and costs only about $15 to $20. So should everyone be tested for it? According to the American Heart Association, the only people who will benefit from CRP testing are those with an intermediate risk of cardiovascular events—that is, a 10% to 20% risk of such events in the next 10 years. (To determine your risk level, ask your doctor or go to the Web site http://hin.nhlbi.nih.gov/atpiii/calculator.asp?usertype=prof.)

For people with an intermediate risk of experiencing a cardiovascular event in the next 10 years, a high CRP level may indicate the need to begin a more intense program of stroke prevention. It may also help motivate people who are at moderate risk for stroke to improve their prevention efforts, such as lowering blood pressure, quitting smoking, and eating healthier.

People already at high risk for cardiovascular events and those with established cardiovascular disease will not benefit from having a CRP test, according to the American Heart Association. Such people should already be aware of their elevated risk, and finding an elevated CRP level will not provide any additional information.

Getting Your Results
If you are at intermediate risk for cardiovascular disease and choose to have a CRP test, you should undergo the test twice—at least two weeks apart—and average the results. (You shouldn't undergo the test if you have an infection or condition that causes inflammation, since it will influence the results.) Be sure to get the high-sensitivity CRP (hs-CRP) test, the only one that can detect small differences in CRP. Note that the CRP test doesn't replace an evaluation for other stroke risk factors, and that an elevated CRP alone does not provide sufficient evidence to warrant the initiation of drug therapy.

Treating High CRP Levels
Currently, no drug is specifically designed to lower elevated CRP levels, and no clinical trial has been conducted to show that lowering CRP reduces the risk of stroke or heart attack. However, if you have a high CRP level, there are numerous ways you can lower it and possibly decrease your risk of cardiovascular disease. These measures are the same as the ones recommended to reduce other risk factors for stroke and heart attack.

Physical activity. A correlational study of 722 men published in *Arteriosclerosis, Thrombosis, and Vascular Biology* in 2002 found that the more men exercised, the lower their CRP levels were. While some preliminary data suggest that initiating a regular exercise program may cut CRP levels by up to 35%, the type and intensity of exercise that may be necessary to reduce CRP have not been established.

Weight. If you are overweight, losing weight may also lower CRP levels. A 2002 *Circulation* report found that CRP levels fell by 32% in 25 obese postmenopausal women who lost an average of 32 lbs.

Aspirin. Aspirin not only reduces the likelihood of a blood clot, but also decreases inflammation, two important factors related to CRP levels. Talk to your doctor before beginning to take aspirin to lower your CRP levels.

Statin drugs. Statin drugs, which lower LDL cholesterol levels, also lower CRP levels. In a 2001 *New England Journal of Medicine* study of 5,742 people with elevated CRP but normal LDL cholesterol levels, those who received lovastatin (Mevacor) reduced their CRP levels by 15%.

However, more definitive data are needed before physicians routinely prescribe statins to lower CRP in people with normal LDL cholesterol levels. Researchers are currently performing such a trial in about 15,000 people, but the results will not be available for a few years.

ACE inhibitors. Some research indicates that ACE inhibitors, a group of antihypertensive drugs, can also decrease CRP levels. But more studies are needed before doctors begin to prescribe ACE inhibitors for people with elevated CRP levels but normal blood pressure.

of atherosclerotic plaque in a brain artery. Between 11% and 30% of TIAs result from emboli originating in the heart.

Accidents and other circumstances. Bone fractures, open heart surgery, the collapse of a lung (a pneumothorax), or too rapid an ascent from deep waters can result in blood clots that can lead to cerebral embolism. A violent blow to the head may cause a hemorrhagic stroke. Mild kidney dysfunction also may raise the risk of stroke.

Risk Factors That Can Be Changed

The following factors raise the risk of stroke; all of them can be minimized or eliminated through lifestyle changes or medical therapy.

Hypertension. High blood pressure, the single greatest risk factor for stroke, is estimated to play a role in about 70% of all ischemic and hemorrhagic strokes. Elevations in either systolic or diastolic blood pressure increase the risk of stroke in both men and women and in people of all ages. Indeed, stroke risk is about four times greater in those with blood pressures of 160/95 mm Hg or above than in those with blood pressures of 140/90 mm Hg or below. A recent meta-analysis concluded that the risk of stroke was increased 10 to 12 times in people with diastolic blood pressures of 105 mm Hg or higher compared with those with diastolic pressures of less than 76 mm Hg.

Cigarette smoking. Smoking is an important contributor to both ischemic and hemorrhagic strokes. A recent meta-analysis found that cigarette smokers have a 50% higher risk of stroke than nonsmokers. The more cigarettes smoked, the greater the risk. Smoking appears to accelerate the progression of atherosclerosis as well as promote the formation of blood clots. Also, nicotine briefly raises blood pressure after each cigarette and causes a buildup of carbon monoxide in the blood that reduces the blood's oxygen-carrying capacity and thus the amount of oxygen available to the brain. Fortunately, the increased risk of stroke associated with smoking decreases after quitting, and the risk returns to normal within five years of smoking cessation.

Diabetes. People with diabetes have a threefold higher risk of ischemic stroke than the general population. Women with diabetes are at greater risk than men. Diabetes is treatable, and evidence is growing that controlling blood sugar may lower stroke risk. Diabetes does not appear to increase the risk of hemorrhagic strokes.

Carotid stenosis. The carotid arteries in the neck supply blood to the brain. If a carotid artery becomes narrowed by the buildup of atherosclerotic plaque, blood flowing through will make an abnormal sound called a bruit. A doctor can hear this sound by placing a stethoscope over the carotid arteries in the neck. When a bruit is heard, especially in people with a history of TIA, a duplex ultrasound (see pages 63–64) is performed to determine the extent of the narrowing. Even in people without a history of TIA, a carotid bruit suggests an increased risk of ischemic stroke since it usually indicates atherosclerotic narrowing of the carotid artery. In general, people with carotid stenosis are three times more likely to

NEW RESEARCH

Smoking Increases Risk of Hemorrhagic Stroke

A new study shows that men who smoke cigarettes have an increased likelihood of having a hemorrhagic stroke, including both intracerebral hemorrhage and subarachnoid hemorrhage.

According to data from more than 22,000 male physicians followed for nearly 18 years, current smokers were 2.4 times more likely to have a hemorrhagic stroke than men who never smoked or had quit smoking. Current smokers had a twofold increased risk of intracerebral hemorrhage and a 3½-fold increased risk of subarachnoid hemorrhage. The rate of hemorrhagic stroke was particularly high in those who currently smoked 20 or more cigarettes a day. Men who had quit smoking and those who never smoked had similar lower rates of hemorrhagic stroke.

Cigarette smoking increases the risk of hemorrhagic and ischemic stroke to a similar degree, the authors say. Smoking likely contributes to hemorrhagic strokes by causing structural damage to the walls of arteries.

"Our results add to the multiple health benefits that can be accrued by abstaining from cigarette smoking," the authors conclude.

STROKE
Volume 34, page 1151
May 2003

suffer a stroke than the general population.

Heart disease. Since many of the same factors contribute to both stroke and coronary heart disease, it is not surprising that the risk of stroke is doubled in those with coronary heart disease. It is uncertain whether treatment of coronary heart disease will prevent strokes, however. Other heart diseases can increase stroke risk by promoting the formation of emboli. These conditions include heart attack, heart failure (impaired ability of the heart to pump blood), valvular heart disease (damage to one or more of the heart's valves), and various cardiac arrhythmias (abnormal heart rhythms), especially atrial fibrillation.

Alcohol abuse. Moderate alcohol consumption (two or fewer drinks per day) is associated with a reduced risk of ischemic stroke. By contrast, even moderate alcohol consumption raises the risk of hemorrhagic stroke. Habitual alcohol intake in excess of two drinks per day almost doubles the risk of stroke by producing abnormal heart rhythms, raising blood pressure, and promoting blood clot formation.

Oral contraceptives and hormone replacement therapy. Older, high-dose estrogen oral contraceptives increased the risk of stroke in women who were over age 35 and smoked cigarettes, had high blood pressure, or had a history of migraine headaches. The low-dose oral contraceptives used today are still associated with a risk of stroke, but the risk is small.

Hormone replacement therapy, in which estrogen is combined with progestin, also increases the risk of stroke. In a randomized, controlled trial called the Women's Health Initiative, published in 2002, postmenopausal women taking estrogen plus progestin had a 40% increased risk of stroke compared with women taking a placebo. The portion of the trial that examined the estrogen-progestin combination has been halted, but a separate part of the trial is still studying the effects of estrogen alone on stroke risk. Hormone replacement therapy with estrogen alone is suitable only for women who have had a hysterectomy, since estrogen without progestin may increase the risk of uterine cancer.

Drug abuse. Stimulants such as cocaine and amphetamines can cause abnormal heart rhythms, heart attacks, and strokes (particularly intracerebral hemorrhage), even in young, healthy first-time users. Intravenous drug use raises the risk of cerebral embolism.

Abnormal lipid levels. High total and low density lipoprotein (LDL, or "bad") cholesterol, high triglycerides, and low HDL ("good") cholesterol contribute to atherosclerosis and coronary

NEW RESEARCH

Increasing Physical Activity Can Add Years to Your Life

An increase in the amount of exercise performed daily—even small increases in walking distance—may lengthen the life span of older women who are sedentary.

Physical activity was assessed initially and after six years in a study of 9,518 women, age 65 and older. Those who increased the distance they walked daily by one mile during the follow-up had a 48% lower risk of death from any cause, a 36% lower risk of death from stroke and heart attack, and a 51% reduced risk of death from cancer compared with women who remained sedentary. And the more the women increased their physical activity, the greater their reduction in cardiovascular mortality during the 12½-year study.

The decreased risk of death associated with increases in physical activity could have resulted from numerous factors, such as a reduction in risk factors for stroke and heart attack, better fitness of the heart and lungs, and fewer falls (and therefore fewer fractures and less physical disability).

Because active women who became sedentary during the study had death rates similar to women who were sedentary throughout the study, the authors conclude that current physical activity, rather than a history of being active, is important in determining the occurrence of events that may shorten a woman's life span.

JOURNAL OF THE AMERICAN MEDICAL ASSOCIATION
Volume 289, page 2379
May 14, 2003

heart disease, and they are important risk factors for stroke as well. A 21-year study of more than 8,000 Israeli men found that those with HDL cholesterol levels below 35 mg/dL had a 32% greater risk of stroke than men with levels above 43 mg/dL. In addition, a study of about 1,500 New York City residents found that people with HDL levels between 35 and 49 mg/dL had a 35% reduction in ischemic stroke risk, compared with those with HDL levels below 35 mg/dL. Reduction of total cholesterol, LDL cholesterol, and triglyceride levels using statin drugs substantially reduced the risk of ischemic stroke in a recent study of 20,000 people.

Sedentary lifestyle. Studies consistently show that regular physical activity lowers the risk of both ischemic and hemorrhagic stroke, possibly by reducing other stroke risk factors, such as obesity and hypertension. In general, people who are physically inactive are almost three times as likely to suffer a stroke than people who exercise regularly.

Obesity. Obesity increases the risk of stroke by 50% to 100%. Although obesity is associated with other risk factors for stroke, such as hypertension and diabetes, it may be an independent risk factor for stroke. Abdominal obesity (a waist circumference of greater than 40 inches in men or 35 inches in women) has an especially strong impact on diabetes and other risk factors for stroke. A recent study found that abdominal obesity was a better predictor of ischemic stroke than BMI—a measure of weight in relation to height (see the sidebar at right).

C-reactive protein. A newly recognized risk factor for stroke is C-reactive protein, a marker for inflammation. Research shows that people with elevated blood levels of C-reactive protein are at increased risk for ischemic stroke, as well as for heart attack. To learn more about this new risk factor, see the feature on pages 46–47.

PREVENTION OF STROKE

The best way to prevent a stroke is to eliminate or minimize as many of the modifiable risk factors as possible. In general, this can be accomplished by losing weight (if necessary), eating a healthy diet, engaging in regular aerobic exercise, and quitting smoking. Medication may also be needed to control blood pressure, blood lipids, diabetes, and coronary heart disease. In addition, antiplatelet therapy, anticoagulants, carotid endarterectomy, or angioplasty and stents may be necessary for people who have already had a stroke or TIA or are at high risk for having a stroke.

NEW RESEARCH

Abdominal Obesity Linked to Risk of Ischemic Stroke

Obesity is a risk factor for coronary heart disease, diabetes, and high blood pressure. Now a study has firmly established a potent relationship between abdominal obesity and ischemic stroke.

Researchers determined the waist-to-hip ratio of 576 individuals who had suffered their first ischemic stroke and 1,142 patients who had never experienced a stroke. Waist-to-hip ratio is a measure of abdominal obesity.

Patients with high waist-to-hip ratios were three times more likely to have an ischemic stroke than those with low waist-to-hip ratios. The association held true for whites, blacks, and Hispanics and was greater in those younger than 65 years of age. The link between ischemic stroke and abdominal obesity was just as strong as its association with blood pressure or diabetes in previous studies.

Abdominal obesity, the researchers concluded, is a better predictor of ischemic stroke risk than body mass index (BMI; a measure of weight in relation to height), especially among younger people. They recommend that stroke prevention programs place greater emphasis on weight loss and preventing obesity.

STROKE
Volume 34, Page 1586
July 2003

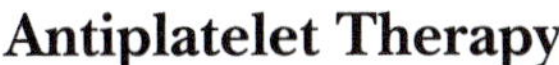

Antiplatelet Therapy

Drugs that reduce blood clot formation by inhibiting the aggregation of platelets in the blood often are prescribed to prevent ischemic strokes in people at high risk, particularly those with asymptomatic carotid bruit or a history of TIA or stroke.

Aspirin. Aspirin is by far the most widely used antiplatelet drug. A recent review of more than 100 clinical trials concluded that aspirin therapy reduces the risk of future strokes by 25% to 30% in people who have had a TIA or minor stroke. (Aspirin is not advised for stroke prevention in otherwise healthy people over age 50 who have not had a stroke or TIA.) Most stroke experts recommend an 81- to 325-mg tablet of aspirin a day to lower stroke risk. People with high blood pressure should lower it before beginning aspirin therapy: A recent study found that the benefits of aspirin in people with high blood pressure are limited mainly to those whose hypertension is under control.

Ticlopidine. Another antiplatelet drug, ticlopidine (Ticlid), is slightly more effective than aspirin in preventing strokes and is less likely to cause gastrointestinal bleeding (aspirin's primary side effect). However, ticlopidine is more costly, and 10% to 20% of people taking it have minor reactions like diarrhea or skin rash.

The most serious potential side effect of ticlopidine is a blood disorder called thrombotic thrombocytopenic purpura, which causes fever, a significant decrease in the number of platelets in the blood, neurological changes, and kidney failure. Although rare, thrombotic thrombocytopenic purpura is fatal in about 30% of cases. Ticlopidine is also associated with neutropenia (depletion of the body's infection-fighting white blood cells). Therefore, careful blood monitoring is necessary, especially in the first three months of treatment. Considering the risks and expense of ticlopidine, many experts recommend it mainly for people who cannot tolerate aspirin or who continue to have TIAs or minor strokes despite aspirin therapy.

Clopidogrel. The antiplatelet drug clopidogrel (Plavix) is another option for people at high risk for a stroke. A three-year study of more than 19,000 people who had suffered a recent stroke or heart attack or had peripheral vascular disease found that 75 mg of clopidogrel per day decreased the combined risk of future stroke, heart attack, or death from vascular disease by 34%, compared with a 25% risk reduction in patients taking 325 mg of aspirin a day. The risk of side effects, including rash, diarrhea, and stomach discomfort, was about the same for both drugs. The risk of thrombotic

NEW RESEARCH

Aspirin Resistance Tied to Strokes, Heart Attacks

Doctors often recommend that people who have had an ischemic stroke or heart attack take a daily aspirin, which may prevent a second cardiovascular event by decreasing the likelihood that platelets will form clots. Now, a study suggests that about 5% of people have platelets that do not respond to aspirin in the same way as they do in the rest of the population. These individuals have an increased likelihood of having a second stroke or heart attack even though they are taking aspirin.

The study enrolled 326 people, average age 60, with cardiovascular disease who were taking 325 mg of aspirin daily. About 5% of the participants were resistant to aspirin's antiplatelet effects. These individuals had nearly three times the risk of death, stroke, or heart attack over a 23-month period than those who were responsive to aspirin (24% vs. 10%).

The test for aspirin resistance used in the study is not widely available, and currently there is no convenient, accurate way to determine who has aspirin resistance. But people who experience a stroke or heart attack while taking aspirin may be aspirin resistant and may benefit from another antiplatelet medication, such as clopidogrel (Plavix) or dipyridamole and aspirin (Aggrenox), according to an accompanying editorial.

JOURNAL OF THE AMERICAN COLLEGE OF CARDIOLOGY
Volume 41, pages 961 and 966
March 19, 2003

Antiplatelet and Anticoagulant Drugs 2004

Drug Type	Generic Name	Brand Name	Average Daily Dosage*	Wholesale Cost (Generic Cost)†
Antiplatelets	aspirin	Aspir-Low	81 to 325 mg	81 mg: $4 (325 mg: $2)
		Aspirtab		325 mg: $1 ($2)
		Bayer		325 mg: $6 ($2)
		Easprin		975 mg: $59 (325 mg: $2)
		Ecotrin		81 mg: $6 (325 mg: $2)
		Halfprin		81 mg: $4 (325 mg: $2)
		St. Joseph		81 mg: $5 (325 mg: $2)
	buffered aspirin	Ascriptin	81 to 325 mg	325 mg: $7 ($2)
		Bufferin		325 mg: $5 ($2)
		Buffinol		325 mg: $2 ($2)
		Magnaprin		325 mg: $4 ($2)
	ticlopidine	Ticlid	500 mg	250 mg: $237 ($150)
	clopidogrel	Plavix	75 mg	75 mg: $406
	dipyridamole and aspirin	Aggrenox	400 mg dipyridamole/ 50 mg aspirin	200 mg/25 mg: $191

* These dosages represent an average range for the prevention of stroke. The precise effective dosage varies from patient to patient and depends on many factors. Do not make any changes in your medication without consulting your doctor.

† Average wholesale prices to pharmacists for 100 tablets or capsules of the dosage strength listed. Costs to consumers are higher. If a generic is available, the price is listed in parentheses. Source: *Red Book, 2003* (Medical Economics Data, publishers).

Advantages	Disadvantages
Aspirin is the most widely used and studied of the antiplatelets. It reduces the risk of stroke in people at high risk, for example, those who have had a previous stroke or transient ischemic attack (TIA) and those who suffer from atrial fibrillation (a heart rhythm abnormality). Aspirin helps to prevent the formation of blood clots by inhibiting the aggregation of blood components called platelets.	Common side effects of aspirin include mild stomach pain, heartburn, indigestion, nausea, and vomiting. Serious side effects include peptic ulcers and gastrointestinal bleeding. Use of aspirin with other nonsteroidal anti-inflammatory drugs (NSAIDs) or with anticoagulant drugs such as warfarin increases the risk of these serious side effects. Contact your doctor if you experience bloody or black, tarry stools; severe stomach pain; or vomiting of blood or substances that resemble coffee grounds.
Ticlopidine reduces the risk of stroke in people who have had a previous stroke or TIA. Research shows that ticlopidine is somewhat more effective than aspirin for reducing stroke risk. Like aspirin, ticlopidine prevents platelet aggregation.	Ticlopidine causes more side effects than aspirin and is generally reserved for people who cannot take aspirin or who experience strokes or TIAs while on aspirin therapy. Common side effects of ticlopidine include diarrhea, indigestion, nausea, skin rash, and mild abdominal pain. Rare but serious side effects include hepatitis and blood disorders such as thrombotic thrombocytopenic purpura and neutropenia. To reduce the risk of these serious side effects, blood tests are required every two weeks during the first three months of therapy. Contact your doctor immediately if you experience bruising or bleeding, particularly bleeding that is difficult to stop; fever, chills, or sore throat; sores, ulcers, or white spots in the mouth; dark or bloody urine; difficulty speaking; pale skin; pinpoint red spots on the skin; seizures; weakness; or yellow skin or eyes. Ticlopidine should be used with caution while taking other medications that reduce blood clotting. These medications include warfarin, aspirin, and other NSAIDs. Ticlopidine should not be taken by people with severe liver disease.
Clopidogrel reduces the risk of stroke in people who have had a previous stroke or heart attack or have other blood circulation problems that can lead to a stroke. Research shows that clopidogrel is somewhat more effective than aspirin for stroke prevention. Clopidogrel is preferred over ticlopidine in people who cannot take aspirin or who have strokes or TIAs while on aspirin therapy, since the risk of thrombotic thrombocytopenic purpura is lower with clopidogrel. Clopidogrel prevents blood clot formation by inhibiting platelet aggregation.	Common side effects of clopidogrel include chest, abdominal, back, or joint pain; red or purple spots on the skin; upper respiratory infections; dizziness; flu-like symptoms; and easy bruising. Contact your doctor immediately if you experience bruising or bleeding, especially bleeding that is difficult to stop. Use of clopidogrel with aspirin or other NSAIDs can increase the risk of gastrointestinal bleeding. Clopidogrel should not be used by people with peptic ulcers.
The combination of dipyridamole and aspirin reduces the risk of stroke in people with a previous stroke or TIA. Research shows that combination therapy is more effective than aspirin alone for reducing stroke risk in people with a previous stroke; however, it is no more effective than aspirin in people who have experienced a TIA. Dipyridamole plus aspirin reduces blood clot formation by inhibiting platelet aggregation.	Common side effects of dipyridamole and aspirin include abdominal pain, nausea, vomiting, diarrhea, headache, heartburn, indigestion, and muscle or joint pain. Gastrointestinal bleeding occurs more often with combination therapy than with aspirin alone. Serious bleeding can also occur when combination therapy is taken with anticoagulant drugs (such as warfarin or heparin) or with NSAIDs. Dipyridamole and aspirin should not be used by people with severe liver or kidney disease.

Antiplatelet and Anticoagulant Drugs 2004 (continued)

Drug Type	Generic Name	Brand Name	Average Daily Dosage*	Wholesale Cost (Generic Cost)†
Anticoagulant	warfarin	Coumadin	2 to 10 mg	4 mg: $83 ($63)

* These dosages represent an average range for the prevention of stroke. The precise effective dosage varies from patient to patient and depends on many factors. Do not make any changes in your medication without consulting your doctor.

† Average wholesale prices to pharmacists for 100 tablets or capsules of the dosage strength listed. Costs to consumers are higher. If a generic is available, the price is listed in parentheses. Source: *Red Book, 2003* (Medical Economics Data, publishers).

thrombocytopenic purpura appears to be lower with clopidogrel than with ticlopidine.

Dipyridamole and aspirin. In 1999, the U.S. Food and Drug Administration approved a new drug for stroke prevention for people who have experienced a previous stroke or TIA. The drug (Aggrenox) contains dipyridamole and aspirin, two antiplatelet agents. In a one-year study of about 6,600 people who had suffered a stroke, a combination of dipyridamole and aspirin was twice as effective as either drug alone in preventing a second stroke, although the overall risk of death was unaffected. Bleeding was more common in patients taking the dipyridamole-aspirin combination than in those taking aspirin alone.

Anticoagulants

Anticoagulant drugs also inhibit blood clot formation but work at a different stage in the clotting process than antiplatelets. Specifically, they interfere with the coagulation cascade and fibrin formation by hindering the activity of certain clot-promoting factors. Anticoagulants are the most effective agents for the prevention of cerebral embolisms, especially those occurring in association with atrial fibrillation.

People with atrial fibrillation who have other risk factors for stroke—age 75 and older, hypertension, and previous stroke or TIA—are typically treated with a long-term, low-dose regimen of

Advantages	Disadvantages
Warfarin reduces the risk of stroke in people with atrial fibrillation, especially those with other risk factors for stroke (for example, age 75 and over, high blood pressure, and previous TIA or stroke). In these individuals, warfarin is considerably more effective than aspirin. Warfarin also is used to prevent stroke in people with heart valve disorders and cardiomyopathy (deterioration of heart muscle). Warfarin prevents strokes by hindering the activity of substances that promote blood clot formation.	Warfarin is associated with a high risk of serious bleeding. To prevent this side effect, patients must undergo regular blood tests to ensure that they are receiving the correct dose. High doses of vitamin K (found in food or dietary supplements) can decrease the effects of warfarin. Thus, foods high in vitamin K (for example, liver, broccoli, cauliflower, and green leafy vegetables) should be eaten in moderation, and you should tell your doctor about any supplements you are taking. Many medications can increase or decrease the effects of warfarin, so be sure to tell your doctor about all the medications you are using. Contact your doctor immediately if you notice any unusual bleeding or bruising. Signs of unusual bleeding include bleeding from the gums, blood in the urine, nosebleeds, pinpoint red spots on the skin, and heavy bleeding from cuts or wounds.

anticoagulant medication, usually warfarin (Coumadin); those with no other risk factors for stroke usually are given aspirin instead. People with heart valve disorders, heart muscle damage from a heart attack, cardiomyopathy (deterioration of heart muscle), or patent foramen ovale (a hole between the left and right sides of the heart) also typically receive warfarin to reduce the risk of cerebral embolism.

Warfarin is associated with a high risk of excessive bleeding. Consequently, people taking warfarin must have regular blood tests to ensure that the dose is correct—high enough to reduce blood clotting, but not so high as to provoke bleeding. The test, called prothrombin time, measures how long it takes for blood to clot. People taking warfarin must also watch their consumption of vitamin K (from both food and supplements), since higher or lower intakes than usual can alter the drug's effectiveness. For more information on using warfarin safely, see the feature on pages 60–61.

Carotid Endarterectomy

When diagnostic imaging tests (see pages 62–64) reveal that one or both carotid arteries in the neck are substantially narrowed by atherosclerotic plaque, a surgical procedure called carotid endarterectomy can be performed to remove the plaque. The procedure takes about two hours and usually requires two to three days of hospitalization.

Carotid endarterectomy significantly reduces the risk of stroke and TIA in some patients. However, it is not appropriate for everyone with carotid stenosis. Long-term results are best for patients who have had a mild stroke or symptoms of a TIA and whose carotid arteries are severely blocked—70% or more. (Completely blocked carotid arteries cannot be reopened, however.) Carotid endarterectomy is not recommended for people with mild blockage (less than 30%).

For people with moderate stenosis (between 30% and 69%), who have had a minor stroke or TIA, carotid endarterectomy may be beneficial, but the degree of benefit is less than that with higher levels of stenosis. A trial called NASCET (North American Symptomatic Carotid Endarterectomy Trial) found that people who underwent carotid endarterectomy for 50% to 69% stenosis had a five-year stroke rate of 16%, compared with a rate of 22% in patients treated with medication alone. In addition, men appeared to benefit more than women, and overall benefits were less in patients at high risk for complications related to the procedure itself. Decisions about whether people with moderate carotid stenosis should undergo carotid endarterectomy are made on a case-by-case basis.

The most recent research suggests that carotid endarterectomy may also benefit people with no symptoms or history of stroke (that is, those with asymptomatic carotid bruit) when blockage of the carotid artery exceeds 60%. In such cases, carotid endarterectomy appears to significantly lower the risk of a first-time stroke in men, but the risk was lowered only minimally in women. (The probable reason for this gender difference is that women are at higher risk for surgical complications because of their smaller arteries.) The reduction in risk, however, is more often for TIAs and minor strokes than for fatal or disabling strokes.

A recent review of 25 studies showed that the overall risk of death or stroke due to carotid endarterectomy was significantly lower for asymptomatic patients than for those with symptoms—3.4% vs. 5.2%. Asymptomatic patients may fare better because the same factors that prevent them from having symptoms (for example, being less prone to blood clots) make them less likely to have complications from carotid endarterectomy. Because the procedure only decreases the overall incidence of stroke in asymptomatic men from 10% to 5%, questions remain about its relative benefits and risks in such patients. These questions are more difficult to answer for women since a recent study found that women with no history of TIA or stroke had a 5.3% risk of stroke or death

Choosing a Surgeon for Carotid Endarterectomy

When considering carotid endarterectomy, the skill and experience of the surgeon, as well as how often the procedure is performed at your hospital, can make a significant difference in the outcome.

For example, in a study of nearly 36,000 carotid endarterectomy patients published in the *Journal of the American College of Surgeons* in December 2002, the risk of death was almost three times higher (1.1% vs. 0.4%) for those treated by surgeons who performed the procedure less than 10 times per year than by surgeons who performed the procedure at least 30 times per year.

Experts recommend that you not only choose a surgeon who performs the procedure frequently, but also seek out a medical center with a complication rate of no more than 3% to 4%—or even 2% to 3% if you have asymptomatic carotid stenosis.

Finding the right surgeon and facility involves research and getting recommendations from other specialists. Here are guidelines and questions to ask that will help you make confident choices.

Questions To Ask	Comments
Is the surgeon a board-certified vascular surgeon or neurosurgeon? What training has he/she had? How many times has he/she performed the surgery? How many operations does he/she do a year?	The goal here is to find a surgeon with plenty of experience. As a general rule, an experienced surgeon will have performed at least 150 carotid endarterectomies, but it's more important that he or she perform at least 12 per year. Preferably, the surgeon should perform the procedure several times a week.
Does the surgeon keep a record of patient outcomes? What percentage of his/her patients have postoperative complications? What percentage have a stroke within five years?	These types of questions should help to reveal the surgeon's skill. Don't be shy about asking for figures: Surgeons expect potential patients to ask for statistics and should have no problem offering this information. If a surgeon is not able to provide numbers or percentages that make you feel comfortable, you may want to look elsewhere.
Does the surgeon specialize in carotid endarterectomy? Does he/she keep updated with the latest in medical technology and research? How does he/she handle specific complications that may arise from the surgery?	Make sure that your surgeon, even if highly experienced, is keeping abreast of advances in his or her specialty. You want to be sure that your surgeon has enough experience to cope with any complications that may arise from the surgery.
Does the surgeon screen patients carefully so that carotid endarterectomy is performed only in those for whom the benefits outweigh the risks?	Carotid endarterectomy is most beneficial in people whose carotid arteries are at least 70% blocked; the procedure may or may not be beneficial in people with 30% to 69% blockage. Carotid endarterectomy is not recommended for people with less than 30% blockage.
Is the medical center where the operation will be performed an accredited and high-volume institution?	Each year, *U.S. News and World Report* publishes a list of the nation's best hospitals. The top 10 hospitals for neurology and neurosurgery are reprinted on page 79.
Do you feel comfortable with your doctor? Can you ask questions and get satisfactory answers? Is the doctor personable and sympathetic?	Do not underestimate the importance of feeling at ease with the surgeon. To have the least stressful experience, you must trust your surgeon. Patients should be involved in their medical treatment and have confidence in their doctors.

during hospitalization after carotid endarterectomy, while men with the same history had only a 1.6% risk.

People with coronary heart disease, uncontrolled diabetes or hypertension, advanced cancer, and serious deficits from a prior stroke may not be able to undergo carotid endarterectomy. Advanced age, however, does not rule out a person as a candidate for surgery: Studies have reported favorable results in people in their 70s and 80s (see the sidebar at right).

Carotid endarterectomy nonetheless is associated with significant risks. The rate of serious complications (such as tearing the carotid artery or triggering a stroke or heart attack) varies with the medical center and the skill of the surgeon but in general ranges between 3% and 15%. By comparison, about 2% of patients have a stroke and 5% to 10% have a heart attack after bypass surgery. Experts recommend that carotid endarterectomy be done by an experienced surgeon at a medical center known to have a complication rate of no more than 3% to 4%. Hospitals that frequently perform carotid endarterectomy (more than 21 procedures per year) tend to have lower complication rates. Getting a second opinion is strongly encouraged before undergoing carotid endarterectomy, especially for asymptomatic patients. For advice on finding a surgeon to perform carotid endarterectomy, see the feature on page 57.

Angioplasty and Stents

Angioplasty involves inflating a small balloon in a blocked artery to enlarge the path for blood flow. The procedure, which was first used in patients with coronary heart disease, has been adopted to reopen partially blocked carotid arteries. Sometimes a stent—a flexible metal tube placed inside a clogged artery to keep it propped open—is implanted during angioplasty. Clinical trials are now under way to compare the results of carotid endarterectomy with those of carotid angioplasty with stenting.

To perform carotid angioplasty with stenting, a radiologist inserts a catheter into an artery in the groin and threads it up into the narrowed portion of the carotid artery. Initially, the stent is collapsed around a deflated balloon at the tip of the catheter. After inflating the balloon to widen the artery, the radiologist expands the stent until it locks in position. The stent acts as a permanent brace inside the artery. It helps maintain blood flow to the brain and may reduce the risk of ischemic stroke.

The results of research on carotid angioplasty with stenting have been mixed, and some researchers have raised concerns about the

NEW RESEARCH

Carotid Endarterectomy Extends Life for Octogenarians

New research shows that carotid endarterectomy can be beneficial for people age 80 and older.

The research—which looked at 1,796 carotid endarterectomies performed in Australia between 1988 and 1998—found that a greater percentage of carotid endarterectomy patients younger than age 80 were alive five years after the operation than those age 80 and older who underwent the procedure (80% vs. 65%). However, people 80 and older who underwent carotid endarterectomy were 18% more likely to survive the next five years than were age-matched controls from the general population. In comparison, carotid endarterectomy patients younger than 80 were 5% less likely to live through the next five years compared with age-matched controls.

One percent of the carotid endarterectomy patients experienced a nonfatal stroke within a month of the surgery, but none of these strokes occurred in patients older than 80.

"The likelihood of living long enough to gain benefit from a carotid endarterectomy was not jeopardized by being too old," the authors conclude. However, the patients who underwent carotid endarterectomy in the study were carefully selected and may not be representative of all octogenarians at risk for stroke.

STROKE
Volume 34, page e95
July 2003

procedure. One major concern is blood clots, which may be released from the carotid artery during the procedure or form on the stent. These clots may travel to an artery in the brain and cause a stroke. Questions also remain about the long-term reliability and structural integrity of stents placed in the carotid arteries, since there is more movement in the neck than around the heart.

For now, carotid angioplasty with stenting may be a good option for high-risk patients with unstable heart conditions who are unable to withstand the rigors of carotid endarterectomy, which is a more extensive surgical procedure. Carotid angioplasty with stenting also may be useful in people who have had a prior carotid endarterectomy, neck surgery, or radiation to the neck area, which increases the risks of carotid endarterectomy.

Researchers are also studying the use of mildly radioactive stents and stents coated with anticoagulant materials or drugs. These innovations may reduce the risk of stroke after angioplasty and eventually allow more widespread use of the technique.

DIAGNOSIS OF STROKE

When a patient arrives at an emergency room with symptoms of a stroke, time is of the essence: Fast action can minimize neurological damage and even mean the difference between life and death. The doctor must rule out other potential causes of the symptoms (such as seizure, brain tumor, diabetic coma, low blood sugar, or migraine headache) and determine the type of stroke (ischemic or hemorrhagic). He or she must also identify what caused the stroke and which part or parts of the brain are affected.

Patient History

A diagnosis of stroke is suspected when a person experiences a loss of one or more brain functions and the symptoms come on suddenly or become apparent on awakening, especially in a person over age 50 with vascular disease or other risk factors for stroke. Although symptoms may progress for a few hours, the condition usually stabilizes within 12 to 24 hours.

If a person with suspected stroke is conscious and able to speak, or if a family member or close friend is present, the doctor will ask questions about the patient's medical background, including any history of TIA, stroke, or recent head injury. The doctor will also ask about the symptoms: what they are, when they started, and how long they have lasted. The patient's age, sex, race, and history of other

NEW RESEARCH

Statins Lower Stroke Risk

Statin drugs reduce the risk not only of heart attacks but also of strokes in people at risk for a heart attack or other coronary event, a new meta-analysis of 38 studies shows.

The meta-analysis revealed that use of a lipid-lowering drug or diet decreased the risk of stroke by 17% in these individuals over nearly a five-year period. However, a specific type of lipid-lowering medication called a statin lowered the stroke risk by 26% during this time. Regardless of the type of lipid-lowering therapy, stroke prevention appeared to be limited to nonfatal strokes.

The advantage of statins over other lipid-lowering drugs in preventing stroke may have resulted from the statins' greater ability to lower cholesterol. Nonstatin lipid-lowering drugs (which include fibrates and bile acid sequestrants) lowered total cholesterol levels by an average of 8%, while statins lowered these levels nearly 22%. Reduction in stroke risk was optimal when total cholesterol dropped below 232 mg/dL.

The meta-analysis combined the results of over 83,000 people who were at high risk for a first or second coronary event. If future studies also show a reduction in stroke risk in people at a high risk for stroke, lipid-lowering drugs like statins may become "essential drugs" for preventing strokes in people who've already had one, the researchers write.

ARCHIVES OF INTERNAL MEDICINE
Volume 163, page 669
March 24, 2003

Using Warfarin Safely

Warfarin can prevent dangerous blood clots that lead to strokes, but it can also carry real risks.

Over the past decade, the number of people taking warfarin (Coumadin) has grown significantly. According to a study published in the *Journal of the American College of Cardiology* in January 2003, doctors prescribed warfarin to 13% of eligible patients with atrial fibrillation in 1990. By 2002, 45% of eligible patients were receiving warfarin. With so many people taking warfarin, and with potentially greater numbers doing so in the future, it is critical that patients understand how to use this medication safely.

What Is Warfarin?

Warfarin is an anticoagulant—a drug that helps prevent the formation and growth of blood clots. It works by blocking the action of vitamin K, which is required to synthesize clotting factors in the liver. These clotting factors are present in the blood and are essential for formation of blood clots. Blood clots in the heart can break loose and block arteries that supply the brain, causing a stroke; blood clots in leg veins can break loose and block arteries that supply the lungs, causing pulmonary embolism.

Warfarin is used for the prevention and treatment of blood clots in people with atrial fibrillation, artificial heart valves, venous thrombosis (clots in the legs), or pulmonary embolism. Doctors sometimes also prescribe warfarin for people who have had a heart attack to decrease their risk of stroke, subsequent heart attack, and death.

What Are the Risks?

Because warfarin reduces blood clotting, its most common side effect is excessive bleeding. The medication has a narrow dosage range in which it is effective at preventing dangerous clots without causing undue bleeding. In addition, many factors can alter warfarin's effects, including age, other medications, current health, medical history, and diet. Therefore, the dosage of warfarin needs to be individualized in each patient to achieve the desired anticlotting effect without increasing the risk of bleeding.

People who take warfarin should always be on the lookout for any signs of excessive bleeding. Conspicuous signs include nosebleeds; cuts that take a long time to stop bleeding; gums that bleed while brushing your teeth; vomiting blood; red or dark brown urine; and black or red stools. Other signs include a sudden onset of weakness, dizziness, or severe headache and unexplained swelling, bruising, or pain. Call your doctor immediately if you notice any of these signs.

Blood Tests

To determine the correct dose of warfarin, periodic blood tests—specifically a prothrombin time (PT) test—are needed to see how quickly the blood clots. If the blood clots too quickly, the dose of warfarin may be increased. If it clots too slowly, the dose may be decreased.

The PT test often involves drawing blood from a vein with a needle, but newer tests need only a small drop of blood that can be obtained with a simple fingerstick. The test is performed every day over the first few days of treatment. Then the test is performed two or three times a week for another week or two. After that, if the results of the PT test are stable over time, a PT test is required only once every four to six weeks.

Because not all laboratories measure PT in the same way, investigators developed a standardized measurement of blood-clotting time called the international normalized ratio (INR). The higher the INR, the slower the clotting time is. The American College of Chest Physicians recommends that most patients have an INR between 2 and 3, a level that is usually effective in preventing dangerous blood clots without causing undue bleeding. However, patients may require a higher INR if they are at particularly high risk for blood clots.

Although health care professionals often perform the PT tests, some of them prescribe home PT tests to their patients. Two home PT tests are available: CoaguChek and ProTime Microcoagulation System. These home tests require a fingerstick to obtain blood, similar to the way in which people with diabetes measure their blood glucose levels. While home testing allows you to monitor your therapy frequently and carefully, detailed instruction in its use is required.

medical conditions (such as diabetes, cardiovascular disease, hypertension, hemophilia, and allergies) also are crucial, and the doctor must know if the patient is taking any medications (prescription, over the counter, or herbal) or illicit drugs.

What Factors Alter Warfarin's Effectiveness?
While numerous factors can increase or decrease warfarin's effects, the two main factors that can be controlled are medication use (prescription, over the counter, or herbal) and diet (specifically, intake of vitamin K).

Medication. Commonly used prescription medications, over-the-counter drugs, and herbal products that may alter warfarin's effects are listed in the inset box at right. This list is not exhaustive, so be sure to tell your doctor about all the medications you are taking before you begin treatment with warfarin. Because your doctor will take your medication use into account when determining the dosage of warfarin you need, you should not alter the dose of or stop taking these other medications without consulting your doctor. You may need more frequent PT tests when starting, stopping, or changing the dosage of these other medications.

Herbal products are a particular concern for people taking warfarin because they are not regulated and each batch may contain different levels of the active ingredient. Also, be aware that alcohol, particularly when used intermittently, can alter warfarin's effects. Therefore, doctors recommend that people avoid alcohol when taking warfarin.

Diet. Vitamin K, either in the diet or in dietary supplements, can interfere with warfarin's anticlotting action. Since your dosage of warfarin takes into account your usual intake of vitamin K, be sure to consume a consistent level of vitamin K from day to day. You will need to be extra careful when you are dieting, feeling ill, or traveling. Foods high in vitamin K include vegetables such as broccoli, spinach, cabbage, Brussels sprouts, and kale; vegetable oils, especially canola and soybean oils; and products that contain the fat substitute olestra (Olean).

Other Ways To Reduce Bleeding Risk
To use warfarin safely, it is extremely important that you take it according to your doctor's instructions. You should also take it at the same time each day. Furthermore, be sure to tell any doctors, pharmacists, nurses, or dentists who treat you that you are taking warfarin. This disclosure is particularly important if you are having surgery or dental work since you may need to temporarily reduce your warfarin dosage or stop taking it altogether a few days before the procedure. Have a discussion with your doctor before stopping any medication. Also, you should avoid any sports or activities that could cause traumatic injury or bleeding.

Products That Can Interact With Warfarin

Here's an overview of some common drugs and other agents that may enhance or reduce warfarin's effectiveness. It is not a complete list.

Products that can enhance warfarin's effects:
- analgesics such as acetaminophen (Tylenol)
- beta-blockers
- oral antidiabetes drugs
- nonsteroidal anti-inflammatory drugs like aspirin (including topical preparations that contain aspirin), ibuprofen (Advil, Motrin, and other brands) naproxen (Aleve and other brands), celecoxib (Celebrex), and rofecoxib (Vioxx)
- garlic
- Ginkgo biloba
- ginseng

Products that can reduce warfarin's effects:
- antacids
- antihistamines
- barbiturates
- immunosuppressive drugs
- St. John's wort

Products that can either enhance or reduce warfarin's effects:
- antibiotics
- antidepressants
- diuretics
- medications to reduce stomach acid—for example, proton pump inhibitors like omeprazole (Prilosec) and H_2 receptor antagonists like cimetidine (Tagamet)
- alcohol

Physical Examination

Along with the patient history, the physician will conduct a general physical examination to check breathing, pulse, blood pressure, and body temperature. The physician can listen for heart rhythm disturbances (such as atrial fibrillation) and for bruits in the carotid arteries. Close examination of the blood vessels in the eyes also is important, since it can reveal evidence of brain hemorrhage, hypertension, emboli, and other conditions related to stroke.

In addition, a neurological examination is done. The doctor will take a quick inventory of the patient's emotional status, memory, motor strength and skills, balance, gait, responsiveness to tactile stimuli, reflexes, vision, eye movements, and speech and language abilities. Deficits in any of these basic neurological functions help the doctor to determine which areas of the brain have been damaged by the stroke.

Laboratory Tests

Blood tests and urinalysis can help the doctor to identify conditions—such as low blood sugar, diabetes, high red blood cell count, an infected heart valve, or syphilis—that can mimic or cause a stroke. Other blood tests that may help pinpoint the cause of a stroke include measurements of blood clotting, platelets, and erythrocyte sedimentation rate. High blood cholesterol levels suggest a possible cerebral thrombosis due to atherosclerosis. An electrocardiogram (ECG or EKG) can detect a heart attack or an abnormal heart rhythm—a potential cause of cerebral embolism.

Imaging Techniques

The most definitive way to diagnose the type of stroke is to locate a blockage in a carotid artery or an artery within the brain, identify the site where damage has occurred in the brain, or detect an abnormal pool of blood within the brain tissue or the subarachnoid space. This can be accomplished with imaging techniques such as computed tomography (CT or CAT) scanning, magnetic resonance imaging (MRI), ultrasound scanning, cerebral angiography, magnetic resonance angiography (MRA), or spiral CT scanning.

Computed tomography (CT or CAT) scans. In this test, the patient lies flat on a special table while x-rays are passed through the body and sensed by a detector that rotates 360° around the patient. A computer combines all the information to create a two-dimensional, cross-sectional picture. CT scans are 10 to 20 times more sensitive than x-rays.

CT scans are most effective for rapidly determining whether an intracerebral or subarachnoid hemorrhage has occurred, as well as to reveal the location and extent of the hemorrhage. Sometimes the scans can detect aneurysms or arteriovenous malformations.

However, damage inflicted by even a large ischemic stroke may not show up on a CT scan until hours or days later, and evidence of small strokes (especially those deep in the brain) may not be visible at all. Therefore, CT scans are not used in the diagnosis of ischemic stroke.

Magnetic resonance imaging (MRI). This technique requires the patient to lie still for 30 minutes or more. Magnetic fields and radio waves are used to generate a three-dimensional image of the brain. An MRI scan is more expensive than a CT scan and is not always practical because of the time required, but it provides clearer pictures and can detect smaller injuries in the brain.

Ischemic strokes may show up on an MRI scan as early as 6 to 12 hours after symptom onset. New developments in MRI technology may allow even earlier detection and the possibility of predicting the size, severity, and reversibility of neurological deficits. For instance, diffusion-weighted MRI can detect injury from an ischemic stroke within one to two hours based on alterations in water movement in the brain; perfusion-weighted MRI can show the degree of blood flow to areas in the brain. Combining diffusion and perfusion imaging may hold the key to determining which patients might benefit from thrombolytic therapy after a stroke.

According to the most recent guidelines from the American Heart Association, an MRI of the brain is not necessary to initiate emergency treatment of a stroke. However, the organization recognizes the existence of special circumstances, and decisions as to whether to perform an MRI scan in a stroke patient should be made on an individual basis.

Ultrasound scanning. Ultrasound scanning uses high-frequency sound waves to generate two-dimensional images of internal body structures. Ultrasound is especially useful for determining the site of an ischemic stroke, since it allows the doctor to visualize blockages and monitor blood flow through specific arteries.

Several ultrasound techniques have been developed and each has its own advantages. Doppler ultrasound generally is used to measure how fast blood is moving through the carotid arteries; a faster flow rate indicates a site where atherosclerotic plaque has narrowed the blood vessel. (Color Doppler Flow Imaging is an enhancement of this technique that uses colors to indicate the speed of blood flow.)

B-mode imaging is another form of ultrasound. It provides a three-dimensional view of the carotid arteries. When combined with Doppler ultrasound, it is known as duplex scanning. Compared with CT scans, MRI scans, and other types of ultrasound

NEW RESEARCH

Silent Strokes Increase Risk of Dementia

Having a symptomatic stroke is known to increase the risk of dementia. Now a study from the Netherlands shows that older people who have had "silent strokes"—that is, strokes that cause no symptoms—are also at an increased risk for dementia.

In the study, researchers performed magnetic resonance imaging (MRI) and tests of cognitive functioning in 1,015 people, age 60 to 90, who did not have dementia and had never had a symptomatic stroke. The same exams were performed four years later to look for evidence of silent strokes and dementia.

Those whose MRI showed evidence of silent strokes at the first exam had a 2.3-fold increased risk of dementia at the second exam. Cognitive decline was most apparent in people who had evidence of silent strokes both before the first exam and between the first and second exams. People with evidence of silent strokes at the first exam but no new ones at the second exam experienced no further decline in cognitive function.

The study's authors speculate that silent strokes may be especially damaging to the brains of people who are already predisposed to conditions like Alzheimer's disease.

THE NEW ENGLAND JOURNAL OF MEDICINE
Volume 348, page 1215
March 27, 2003

scans, duplex scanning provides the most accurate images of the carotid arteries. Transcranial Doppler scanning may allow an assessment of blood flow through the arteries within the brain.

Cerebral angiography. This procedure involves the insertion of a catheter into the carotid artery and injection of an iodine-based contrast solution into the artery through the catheter. The dye helps produce a high-quality x-ray image of the blood vessels within the brain. Angiography provides more detailed information about blood vessels than the other diagnostic imaging techniques, but because of the risk of complications, it is used only when noninvasive tests prove inadequate. Possible complications include a dangerous allergic reaction to the iodine in the contrast solution, reversible neurological deficits, and a stroke that results in permanent deficits. These complications occur in less than 1% of patients younger than 50 years old, but their incidence rises with age and the presence of hypertension or vascular disease.

Magnetic resonance angiography (MRA). This technique is a refinement of MRI that involves the injection of a weakly magnetic contrast dye into a vein in the arm. The procedure adds about 15 minutes to a conventional MRI scan. MRA has not been perfected but is used increasingly as a screening test for blockage of large vessels. People with a normal MRA may not need to undergo cerebral angiography.

Spiral CT scanning. Spiral CT scanning is a new method of looking at blood vessels. An iodine-based dye is injected into a vein and images of the area of interest are taken as a special table slides through the scanning unit. Computer-based imaging software then isolates the blood vessels that fill with dye. The resulting image resembles that obtained from cerebral angiography and can be rotated and manipulated in three dimensions to look for aneurysms or narrowings. This technique cannot be used in people who are allergic to iodine or have kidney dysfunction.

ACUTE TREATMENT OF STROKE

Immediate emergency care for a stroke requires treatment in a hospital, where life support systems are available (if needed) to maintain breathing and heart function. The specific treatment received depends on whether the stroke is ischemic or hemorrhagic. In an ischemic stroke, the primary goal is to restore or at least improve blood flow to the brain; the goal in a hemorrhagic stroke is to relieve pressure on the brain and stop the bleeding.

Treatment of Ischemic Stroke

Careful monitoring and control of blood pressure are essential after an ischemic stroke. In general, elevated blood pressure is acceptable, since it promotes blood flow through the partially blocked arteries so that blood can reach the jeopardized regions of the brain. The exception is when blood pressure is so high that it is likely to damage the brain, heart, or kidneys. In such cases, it is lowered slowly. Otherwise, efforts are aimed at preventing low blood pressure (hypotension), which can limit the amount of blood reaching the brain. When low blood pressure occurs—whether due to antihypertensive drugs, dehydration, or other causes—it can be treated with intravenous saline solutions to increase blood volume and with blood pressure-raising drugs if needed.

Body temperature also must be carefully monitored and controlled, since fever can worsen damage to the brain. A study of people with stroke found that for every 2.7° F increase in body temperature the risk of a poor outcome (death or a more severe stroke) more than doubled. In fact, deliberately lowering the body temperature of people suffering from a stroke is being examined as a treatment option. For more information about this experimental treatment, see the feature on pages 66–67.

Intravenous fluids containing glucose are usually avoided since excessive glucose in the brain may be detrimental (this practice is controversial, however). Buildup of fluid in the brain (cerebral edema) also can cause damage. Cerebral edema can be treated by limiting fluid intake and raising the head of the patient's bed to a 30° angle.

Drug therapy. Until recently, doctors could do little to intervene while an ischemic stroke was in progress. However, with the approval of the emergency stroke drug, alteplase (Activase), doctors now have a specific course of action to follow for an ischemic stroke. Alteplase, which is also called tissue-type plasminogen activator (t-PA), belongs to a class of drugs known as thrombolytic ("clot-busting") agents.

Thrombolytic drugs have been used widely to treat heart attacks; prompt intravenous administration of alteplase can dissolve a clot that is blocking blood flow to the heart, thereby preventing extensive tissue damage. Some (but not all) studies have shown similar results with alteplase for strokes. But treatment with alteplase causes cerebral hemorrhage (excessive bleeding in the brain) in about 6% of stroke patients.

Early treatment with alteplase is essential. The American Heart

NEW RESEARCH

Coronary Heart Disease Common in Stroke Patients

People who have had a transient ischemic attack (TIA) or ischemic stroke should be evaluated for asymptomatic coronary heart disease (CHD), according to a joint statement from the American Heart Association and the American Stroke Association.

The organizations came to this conclusion after an extensive review of the medical literature on stroke and CHD. They found that about 20% to 30% of people who have an ischemic stroke test positive for CHD, and some 2% to 5% of ischemic stroke patients die of CHD within three months of their stroke. CHD is more likely to be found in patients with ischemic than hemorrhagic strokes, because atherosclerosis is a causative factor in both CHD and ischemic stroke.

Doctors should evaluate the 10-year risk of CHD in people who have had a TIA or stroke, the statement says. People with a 20% or greater risk of CHD should then undergo a noninvasive diagnostic test, such as an exercise stress test, soon after leaving the hospital for the stroke. Those who test positive for CHD should then receive treatment with medication, angioplasty, or bypass surgery.

CIRCULATION
Volume 108, page 1278
September 9, 2003

On the Horizon: Cooling Therapy for Stroke

Inducing mild hypothermia in people who are having a stroke may lessen brain damage.

Despite advances in the treatment of stroke in the past quarter century, physicians are still searching for ways to improve the outcomes of stroke patients. One promising new treatment is mild hypothermia, which involves cooling patients soon after the onset of a stroke.

Research has shown that controlling fever in stroke patients improves outcomes. And now, animal studies and preliminary research in humans suggest that deliberately lowering the body temperature of patients suffering from a stroke, even if they don't have a fever, may help minimize brain damage and widen the "window of opportunity" for treatments like tissue-type plasminogen activator (t-PA). So how might this technique benefit stroke patients, and how does it work?

The Evidence

Investigators first began looking into the benefits of hypothermia in the 1950s, when research revealed that low body temperatures allowed animals to survive with decreased blood flow to the brain during hibernation. Later, in the 1990s, animal studies showed that lowering body temperature decreased the area of the brain that was damaged by a stroke. Hypothermia also appeared to slow or halt the damage that resulted from disrupting oxygen supply to the brain.

More recent studies in humans have demonstrated the safety and feasibility of using hypothermia to treat stroke. One study, published in the *Journal of Neurological Anesthesiology*, looked at the effect of a water-cooled mattress in 18 stroke patients. Doctors were able to keep all but one of the patients' body temperatures below normal for 24 hours, while using drugs to control shivering and other side effects of cooling. Although 61% of the patients experienced side effects (such as vomiting, low blood pressure, and pneumonia), only 12% died within three months of the stroke, compared with 17% in another study that used t-PA.

How Is Cooling Done?

There are numerous ways doctors can slightly lower the body temperature of someone who's experiencing a stroke.

Surface cooling can be done by rubbing a patient's skin with ice bags, ice water, or other cool liquids. Cooling blankets, water-cooled mattresses, and cold air are also effective. These techniques can only be used in a hospital. But researchers are testing a cooling helmet that circulates cool air over the top of the head and neck and can be placed on a patient in an ambulance. Similar helmets were used to keep soldiers cool in the desert heat during the 1991 Gulf War, and the military continues to use an updated version of the device.

Intravascular cooling involves cooling the body from the inside. One approach is to infuse cool fluids into the body intravenously. Another method, called the Celsius Control System, was approved by the U.S. Food and Drug Administration in Janu-

Association recommends in its guidelines that alteplase be used only when it can be given within three hours of the onset of an ischemic stroke. If too much time has elapsed, cerebral hemorrhage may be more likely, and it may be too late to prevent brain damage.

Before receiving alteplase, all patients must have a neurological examination and a CT scan to ensure they are good candidates. Only hospitals equipped for immediate treatment of excessive bleeding should administer alteplase. In addition, alteplase cannot be used in certain individuals, including those who are having a hemorrhagic stroke, have had a stroke in the past three months, have a blood pressure reading greater than 185/110 mm Hg, or are currently taking warfarin or heparin.

For people with stroke due to cerebral embolism, the anticoagulant drug heparin often is administered intravenously for several

ary 2003. With this system, doctors insert a closed catheter into the inferior vena cava (a large vein that passes through the abdomen). A temperature-controlled saline solution is passed though the catheter, and heat exchange occurs when the blood comes in contact with the catheter's tip. The change in the temperature of the blood affects the temperature of organs throughout the rest of the body, including the brain.

How soon to begin cooling, for how long, and to what temperature are still matters of debate. Current evidence seems to indicate that cooling should begin within 6 hours, but not more than 12 hours, after stroke onset. The cooling should last for at least 6 hours, experts say, but the best outcomes appear to occur in patients whose body temperatures are lowered for 24 to 48 hours.

Lower temperatures appear more effective for stroke patients, but they are associated with greater side effects. "Mild" hypothermia—a body temperature between 93.2° and 96.8° F—may be best for people with mild or moderate strokes. "Moderate" hypothermia—89.6° to 93.2° F—may be required for those with severe strokes.

How Cooling Improves Outcomes

Researchers are not entirely sure why cooling may help improve outcomes in stroke patients. Many experts suspect that a major benefit is from the prevention of reperfusion injury, the wave of free-radical formation and brain-cell death that occurs when blood begins flowing again to the deprived area after a stroke. Preventing reperfusion injury also avoids the breakdown of the blood-brain barrier—the layer of cells that block entry of potentially damaging chemicals in the blood into the brain.

Cooling can also prevent the accumulation of fluid in the brain (cerebral edema) and can slow cells' metabolic processes. Further, cooling can be used along with t-PA and may prevent some of its side effects.

Side Effects

Major side effects of cooling patients are discomfort and shivering, which can be minimized with sedatives and sometimes with drugs that cause temporary paralysis. (These side effects are less likely with intravascular than surface cooling, since with intravascular cooling only the internal organs are cooled and the skin remains warm.) Other potential side effects include a drop in blood volume, abnormal heart rhythms, too high or too low blood pressure, pneumonia, increased pressure in the skull, longer blood clotting times, kidney failure, and decreased immune function. Generally, these side effects increase with lower temperatures and are reversed when the patient is rewarmed.

The Bottom Line

To date, no randomized, controlled trials have demonstrated that therapeutically induced hypothermia is an effective treatment for people who've recently suffered a stroke. Nonetheless, the American Stroke Association reported in 2003 that inducing mild hypothermia is a "promising form of neuroprotection" after a stroke. In addition, a number of research groups are currently testing the treatment in randomized trials. If the results of these studies are favorable, cooling may one day become part of standard care for stroke patients.

days to prevent new clots from forming and to keep existing clots from getting any larger. Heparin is also typically used as an immediate treatment for strokes due to severe stenosis in the carotid, vertebral, or basilar arteries (which branch off from the vertebral arteries), although its effectiveness in these situations is not clearly established. Heparin should not be given to people at risk for hemorrhage, for example, those with uncontrolled hypertension, gastrointestinal bleeding, or thrombocytopenia (a low number of blood platelets).

The anticoagulant drug warfarin often is started at the same time as heparin to treat cerebral embolism. Unlike heparin, it can be prescribed in pill form for long-term use; similar to heparin, it should not be given to people at high risk for hemorrhage. In addition, long-term use of warfarin requires careful evaluation. Although the short-term risks from warfarin are small, the chance of complications accumulates over the years. Doctors also must consider whether patients are at risk for falls, since falling and hitting the head could lead to serious bleeding in the brain.

If patients cannot be given warfarin or heparin, aspirin is the next most effective therapy to reduce the risk of future strokes. Patients who experience TIAs or new strokes while on aspirin therapy or experience intolerable side effects can be treated with other antiplatelet agents, such as dipyridamole and aspirin, clopidogrel, or ticlopidine (see pages 51–54).

Another option for the emergency treatment of an ischemic stroke is the administration of a thrombolytic drug directly into the blocked artery. A study of 180 patients looked at intra-arterial administration of a thrombolytic drug called prourokinase within six hours of the onset of an ischemic stroke. Patients received either prourokinase plus heparin or heparin alone. After three months, 40% of the people treated with prourokinase and 25% of those in the heparin-only group were able to function independently. Prourokinase did not decrease the risk of death, however, and people who received the drug had a higher rate of cerebral hemorrhage.

Patients with cerebral embolism due to atrial fibrillation may be treated with antiarrhythmic medications such as amiodarone (Cordarone) and procainamide (Procan, Pronestyl, and other brands). Also, digoxin (Lanoxin), calcium channel blockers, or beta-blockers may be given to keep the heart's ventricles (lower chambers) from responding to the rapid signals from the atria. A rapid ventricular rate can lead to poor cardiac output, low blood pressure, poor blood flow through narrowed arteries in the brain, and heart failure.

Researchers are interested in developing drugs known as cytoprotective (cell-preserving) agents, some of which are designed to prevent or halt the ischemic cascade—the chain of chemical reactions that occurs during an ischemic stroke. Studies of various cytoprotective drugs are currently under way, but the results so far have not been promising.

Surgery. Surgery is rarely part of the immediate treatment of ischemic stroke, although carotid endarterectomy (see pages 55–58) sometimes is performed to treat minor strokes and prevent additional ones in people with severe carotid stenosis. In the aftermath of a large ischemic stroke, the brain needs to time to recover before carotid endarterectomy can be performed. In such cases, surgery may be postponed for as long as six weeks after the stroke. Angioplasty with or without stenting (see pages 58–59) is being used more often, especially in people for whom carotid endarterectomy presents too great a risk.

Treatment of Hemorrhagic Stroke

Because hemorrhagic strokes often occur in association with extremely high blood pressure, the first step in treatment is to lower blood pressure to minimize the amount of bleeding from the ruptured artery. Lowering of blood pressure is done carefully and slowly, since additional brain damage can occur when blood pressure is too low.

Drug therapy. Mannitol (a type of sugar) and diuretics, which reduce fluid retention by increasing sodium and water loss in the urine, can be used to treat cerebral edema (swelling of tissues in the brain), a serious and relatively common consequence of a hemorrhagic stroke. Nimodipine (Nimotop), a calcium channel blocker, may reduce brain damage due to vasospasm (spasm of blood vessels in the brain). Vasospasm often occurs in the first two weeks after a subarachnoid hemorrhage; it further reduces blood flow to the brain and can be fatal.

Surgery. Surgical intervention is warranted in some cases of hemorrhagic stroke, such as those associated with aneurysms or arteriovenous malformations in which there is a high risk of rebleeding. Depending on its location in the brain, an aneurysm that has leaked or ruptured can be clipped across its neck. This procedure stops blood flow into the aneurysm, thus preventing any future bleeding. A newer procedure in which a platinum coil is fed into the aneurysm, sealing it off from blood circulation, is sometimes tried in people who are unable to undergo clipping.

The risk of treating an arteriovenous malformation must be balanced against the possibility of future bleeding, which is minimal in people without symptoms. If a hemorrhage occurs, patients have about a 2% to 3% annual risk of further bleeding. When bleeding occurs from a small arteriovenous malformation, the chance of dying is about 15%. Therefore, the risk of intervention must be lower than this level; if it is not, the arteriovenous malformation usually is monitored closely and the need for treatment reconsidered if the patient's condition worsens.

The three methods of treating an arteriovenous malformation are surgical removal, embolization, and radiation therapy. Which method is employed depends on the position of the arteriovenous malformation (for example, whether it is near any vital structures), its size, its accessibility, and the life expectancy of the patient. A

NEW RESEARCH

Falls After Stroke Often Occur While Dressing

Common risk factors for falls in older people include balance problems, sedative use, previous falls, and incontinence. For women who have had a stroke, the strongest predictor of falls is balance problems while dressing, according to a recent international study.

More than 120 women participated in the study. Half were over age 76, and none were living in a nursing home after their stroke.

The study found that women with a balance problem while dressing had a sevenfold increased risk of falling in the year after having a stroke. In addition, symptoms of general balance difficulties, spinning sensations, and dizziness related to the stroke increased the risk of falling by more than fivefold.

These results indicate stroke patients need to take special precautions to prevent falls, particularly when dressing. These individuals should be seated while dressing, especially when putting on pants, and should wear clothes that are simple to take off and put on. The risk of falls while dressing may be high for stroke patients because of the complicated motions, coordination, and balance that are involved. Falls are an important concern for people on warfarin, who can experience bleeding in the brain if a fall results in head trauma.

STROKE
Volume 34, page 494
February 2003

Relief for Caregivers

Taking care of someone who has had a stroke can be rewarding but tiring. Respite care programs can provide caregivers with a much needed break.

Caring for a stroke survivor at home can be physically and emotionally draining. Respite care, which offers caregivers a temporary break from their duties, can be an invaluable resource. In fact, caregivers who use respite care are able to keep their loved one at home longer than people who do not use this service. In addition, such caregivers often are healthier and feel happier about their caregiving role.

Types of Respite Care

Often, a good way to take a break from caregiving is to have someone you know stay with the person. For those unwilling or unable to rely on family, friends, or neighbors for help, several professional services are available. A few are free, but most involve fees and are not covered by Medicare. The most common types of respite care are in-home care and adult day care.

In-home care involves someone coming to the stroke patient's home to provide companion services, personal care, or household help. In-home care providers can be hired privately, through an agency, or through a government program.

Adult day care offers structured programs in a group setting. These programs are usually held in a community center or facility. The services offered may include transportation to and from the program, lunch, exercise, crafts, discussion, and music. Adult day care may be available from one to five days a week, and a few programs have evening and weekend hours. In general, two types of day care are available: adult social day care provides activities, meals, and some health services, while adult health day care is for people with more severe medical problems who need intensive health assistance.

How To Find Respite Care

A good place to start is your local office on aging, which is usually listed in the government section of the telephone directory. (Note: The actual name of the agency varies from area to area.) Also, the American Stroke Association (see page 78 for contact information) and the organizations listed in the inset box on the opposite page can refer you to groups and services in your area.

What To Look For

Most referral services do not know the quality of the programs they recommend. So when looking for respite care, you need to do your own research and ask questions. Most respite care providers are reputable, but it is important to be alert to any problems.

Here are a few things to ask a potential in-home care provider:

- Have you had special training and

relatively accessible arteriovenous malformation may be removed surgically, while one positioned deep within the brain might be treated with either embolization or radiation therapy.

Embolization involves passing a catheter through the arteries and into the center of the arteriovenous malformation. A "glue" is fed slowly through the catheter and injected into the arteriovenous malformation to fill it. When the glue solidifies, blood flow through the arteriovenous malformation is blocked. Embolization often is done prior to surgical removal of an arteriovenous malformation. Radiation therapy causes the abnormal blood vessels in the arteriovenous malformation to be reabsorbed by the body over a period of a few years.

Hemorrhagic strokes often result in an intracerebral hematoma—a pool of blood within the brain that damages brain cells and can increase pressure within the brain to dangerous levels. (In fact, large hematomas are usually fatal.) Emergency drainage of a

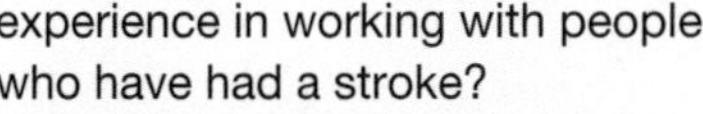

experience in working with people who have had a stroke?

- Are you certified by the state (if applicable)?
- Do you have references?
- What times are you available?
- Who will substitute if you cannot come to work?
- How can I reach your supervisor if I have a concern?
- Can I see how you interact with the stroke patient?

The following are some questions to ask a potential adult day care service:

- Is the staff continually trained in patient care?
- How much supervision is provided?
- What kind of activities do you provide?
- How are meals prepared?
- What kind of fire emergency plan is in place?

Resources for Finding Respite Care

Eldercare Locator
927 15th St. NW, 6th Fl.
Washington, DC 20005
☎ 800-677-1116
www.eldercare.gov

National Council on the Aging
300 D St. SW, Ste. 801
Washington, DC 20024
☎ 202-479-1200
www.ncoa.org

Family Caregiver Alliance
690 Market St., Ste. 600
San Francisco, CA 94104
☎ 415-434-3388
www.caregiver.org

National Adult Day Services Association
8201 Greensboro Dr., Ste. 300
McLean, VA 22102
☎ 866-890-7357
www.nadsa.org

American Association of Retired Persons
601 E St. NW
Washington, DC 20049
☎ 800-424-3410
www.aarp.org

Adjusting to Respite Care

Stroke survivors will need some time to adjust to a new caregiver, especially if you have been providing all or most of their care. Most people respond best if they first have a brief meeting at home with the in-home care provider or someone from the day care center. If possible, schedule this visit at a time when the person is normally calm and feeling well.

You should remain close by during the first few sessions of respite care to help reassure the person that everything is fine. But after that, you should resist the urge to stay. If you are finding this difficult, try leaving for a short time—go visit a friend or take a walk. Feelings of guilt about leaving your loved one are common, but remember that getting some rest will help you be a better caregiver. In addition, the person may enjoy and benefit from spending time with other people.

hematoma, known as evacuation, can relieve the excess pressure and minimize brain damage. Sometimes, however, the hematoma is not accessible, or the release of pressure may result in further bleeding. Blood that seeps into the subarachnoid space or into the cavities within the brain known as the ventricles eventually is reabsorbed into the body. In some people, however, clotted blood interferes with this fluid resorption, leading to an excessive accumulation of fluid (called hydrocephalus or "water on the brain"). Surgery then may be needed to drain the fluid through a tube.

STROKE REHABILITATION

The process of rehabilitation after a stroke starts almost immediately after admission to the hospital and often continues for at least one to two months afterward. At first, the main goal is to reduce or prevent stroke complications, such as stiffening of the limbs and deep vein thrombosis. As the patient's condition stabilizes, the focus turns to longer-term goals of restoring mental and physical function, adapting to disability, returning to an active life, and preventing additional strokes.

Although the exact approach to rehabilitation depends on the specific loss of function caused by the stroke, it typically consists of learning strategies to overcome any deficits and performing exercises to improve range of motion in joints, strengthen weak muscles, and restore function to the greatest extent possible.

The Agency for Health Care Policy and Research has made several recommendations to help patients get the most out of rehabilitation. These include beginning rehabilitation as soon as possible after a stroke, selecting the most appropriate program (inpatient, outpatient, or home based), setting realistic goals (to avoid frustration), frequently assessing progress, and following up during the transition back to the community (when the family plays a major role). Individuals may need to accept some degree of disability, but optimal recovery depends on a combination of the following factors: the patient's determination to succeed, the support of family and friends, and the well-integrated efforts of specialists.

A variety of specially trained professionals are involved in the rehabilitation process. Occupational therapists teach patients new ways to perform day-to-day activities (writing, bathing, cooking, or job-related tasks) affected by their disability. Physical therapists provide instruction and exercises to help patients regain the ability to walk and move about independently, as well as to improve strength, flexibility, balance, and overall fitness. Social workers can provide information on community services available to stroke survivors and their families. Speech-language pathologists help patients regain as much of their lost swallowing ability and language skills as possible.

The eventual goal of any rehabilitation program is for the patient to return to the community, and certain steps must be taken before this transition can be made. Most patients are not fully independent when they first leave a rehabilitation program, so they and their families should be prepared to continue rehabilitation at home. In addition, the patient's home must be made ready for any special needs. It is particularly important that patients and the family members involved in their care understand what to expect and what will be required of them. Doctors and therapists can offer guidance on these issues and discuss what community services are available. A valuable community service for caregivers is respite care—either in-home care or adult day care—which allows caregivers to take a break from their responsibilities (see the feature on pages 70–71).

Because long-term medical treatment after a stroke is complicated, one doctor should be selected to oversee the patient's care. This approach will ensure there are no gaps in treatment and allow for frequent assessments of progress and an eventual phasing out of rehabilitation when patients have progressed as far as they can. Throughout the poststroke period, all medications must be carefully monitored. For example, anticonvulsants or benzodiazepines could affect the ability to participate in rehabilitation exercises and activities.

In general, the best candidates for rehabilitation have at least one significant disability (such as paralysis or aphasia), are moderately stable medically, have the physical endurance to sit up for at least one hour, and are able to learn and participate to some extent in active rehabilitation treatments. However, rehabilitation may be either unnecessary or unfeasible in some cases—for example, for patients who have no disability or are too disabled to benefit. Patients with severe disabilities may be able to begin rehabilitation after a period of rest. ■

GLOSSARY

abulia—Reduction in speech, movement, thought, and emotional reaction as a result of damage to the frontal lobe.

ACE inhibitors—Drugs that lower blood pressure by preventing the formation of angiotensin II, a hormone that causes arteries to constrict and triggers the release of aldosterone. Also used to slow the progression of kidney disease.

agnosia—Loss of the ability to interpret incoming visual, auditory, or tactile stimuli, even though the senses of vision, hearing, and touch are mechanically intact and function normally. Results from damage to the parietal lobe.

aldosterone—A hormone released by the adrenal glands that increases blood pressure by signaling the kidneys to retain sodium, which increases blood volume.

aldosterone blockers—Drugs that lower blood pressure by interfering with the activity of the hormone aldosterone.

aldosteronism—An overproduction of aldosterone caused by a tumor or overgrowth of cells in the adrenal gland. Aldosteronism can lead to hypertension.

alpha-blockers—Drugs that decrease blood pressure by blocking nerve impulses that constrict small arteries.

alteplase—A drug used to treat heart attacks and strokes that works by dissolving blood clots. Also called tissue-type plasminogen activator (t-PA).

ambulatory blood pressure monitor—A portable device that automatically measures and records blood pressure over a 24- to 48-hour period. Measurements are taken while the person goes about daily activities, as well as during sleep.

aneroid blood pressure monitor—A manually operated monitor that consists of a cuff, bulb, and dial gauge to register blood pressure levels.

aneurysm—A ballooning of the wall of a blood vessel caused by weakening of the wall.

angina—Episodes of chest pain caused by an inadequate supply of oxygen and blood to the heart. It occurs most often during physical activity. Also called angina pectoris.

angioplasty—A procedure in which a small balloon is inflated in a blocked artery to enlarge the path for blood flow.

angiotensin—A hormone that has two forms: angiotensin I and angiotensin II. The latter raises blood pressure by causing arteries to constrict and triggering the release of aldosterone.

angiotensin II receptor blockers—Drugs that help lower blood pressure by interfering with the action of angiotensin II, a hormone that causes arteries to constrict and triggers the release of aldosterone.

anticoagulants—Anticlotting drugs that work by inhibiting the formation of fibrin, a protein required for blood clot development. Examples are heparin and warfarin.

antiplatelets—Anticlotting drugs that work by inhibiting the clumping of blood cells called platelets. One example is aspirin.

aphasia—Difficulty in comprehending or producing spoken or written language. Results from damage to the frontal lobe, temporal lobe, or a part of the limbic system called the thalamus.

arrhythmia—An abnormal heart rhythm.

arteriovenous malformation—A disorder present at birth and characterized by a complex, tangled web of arteries and veins.

aspiration pneumonia—Pneumonia caused by the inhalation of food and other particles into the lungs.

atherosclerosis—The narrowing of arteries by fatty deposits (called plaques) within the artery walls that can cause a reduction in blood flow.

atrial fibrillation—A common abnormal heart rhythm in which the heart contracts at a fast and chaotic rate.

atrial natriuretic factor—A hormone produced by the atria of the heart that helps regulate blood pressure by causing the kidneys to excrete more sodium and by inhibiting the production of aldosterone and renin.

baroreceptors—Special nerve endings in the walls of arteries that monitor blood pressure.

beta-blockers—Drugs that impede the actions of epinephrine and norepinephrine, slow heart rate, and lower blood pressure by diminishing cardiac output.

b-mode imaging—An imaging technique that uses high-frequency sound waves to produce a three-dimensional view of the carotid arteries.

brain stem—An area located at the base of the brain above the spinal cord that maintains basic life support functions such as breathing, heart rate, and blood pressure.

calcitriol—A hormone formed from dietary vitamin D that increases the absorption of calcium from the intestine and plays a role in the regulation of blood pressure by constricting small arteries.

calcium channel blockers—Drugs that lower blood pressure by dilating arteries and, in some cases, by decreasing cardiac output.

cardiac output—The amount of blood pumped by the heart.

cardiovascular disease—Disease affecting the arteries that supply blood to the heart and other organs. Coronary heart disease, strokes, and peripheral vascular disease are the most common cardiovascular diseases.

carotid arteries—Blood vessels that carry oxygenated and nutrient-rich blood from the heart to the brain. There are two carotid arteries—one on each side of the front of the neck.

carotid endarterectomy—A surgical procedure to remove plaque from the carotid arteries.

carotid stenosis—A narrowing of the carotid arteries by atherosclerotic plaque.

central alpha agonists—Drugs that lower blood pressure by blocking nerve impulses that constrict small arteries.

cerebellum—The area of the brain located above the brain stem that controls coordination, balance, and posture.

cerebral angiography—A procedure involving the injection of an iodine-based contrast solution into the bloodstream to produce high-quality x-ray images of the blood vessels within the brain.

cerebral edema—Swelling of the brain due to bleeding, trauma, stroke, or a tumor.

cerebral embolism—A blockage of blood flow that occurs when part of a blood clot or a piece of atherosclerotic plaque breaks off and travels through the bloodstream until it lodges in an artery supplying blood to the brain.

cerebral thrombosis—A blockage of blood flow that occurs when a blood clot forms at the site of atherosclerotic plaque within the wall of a major artery supplying the brain. The most common cause of an ischemic stroke.

cerebrum—The largest portion of the brain. It controls conscious thought, perception, voluntary movement, and integration of sensory input.

combination therapy—A treatment approach that uses medication from two or more drug classes.

computed tomography (CT or CAT) scan—A test in which a patient lies flat on a table while x-rays are passed through the body and sensed by a rotating detector. A CT scan of the head can reveal strokes, hemorrhages, and tumors.

coronary heart disease—A narrowing of the coronary arteries by atherosclerosis. Reduces or completely blocks blood flow to the heart. Also called coronary artery disease.

Cushing's syndrome—A condition resulting from the secretion of excessive amounts of cortisone and related hormones by a tumor in the adrenal gland. A potential cause of high blood pressure.

cytoprotective drugs—A class of drugs that protect healthy tissue, for example, during an ischemic stroke.

deep vein thrombosis—The formation of a blood clot in the legs.

diabetes—A disorder characterized by abnormally high levels of glucose (sugar) in the blood.

diastolic blood pressure—The lower number in a blood pressure reading. Represents pressure in the arteries when the heart relaxes between beats.

direct vasodilators—Antihypertensive drugs that act directly on the smooth muscle of small arteries, causing them to widen.

diuretics—A class of drugs that increases loss of sodium through the kidneys, thereby increasing the production of urine and decreasing blood volume and blood pressure.

Doppler ultrasound—The use of sound waves to measure how fast blood moves through arteries, such as the carotid arteries.

electronic blood pressure monitor—A battery-operated blood pressure monitor that uses a microphone to detect blood pulses in an artery. Consists of an inflatable cuff and a gauge with a digital screen.

embolus—A blood clot or a piece of atherosclerotic plaque that travels through the bloodstream until it lodges in a narrowed vessel and blocks blood flow. The plural form is emboli.

endothelin—A hormone that causes blood vessels to constrict.

epinephrine—A hormone that increases blood pressure in response to stress. Also called adrenaline.

frontal lobe—An area at the front of the brain that deals with speech, personality, and motor function.

glomeruli—Sites in the kidneys where blood is filtered and waste products are removed.

glutamate cascade—See **ischemic cascade**.

hematoma—A mass of clotted blood that forms as a result of a ruptured blood vessel.

hemianopia—A condition, often caused by a stroke, that results in blindness on only one side of a person's field of vision in both eyes.

hemorrhagic stroke—A stroke that occurs when an artery in the brain suddenly bursts and blood leaks into the surrounding tissue.

high density lipoprotein (HDL)—A particle in the blood that can protect against coronary heart disease by removing cholesterol from the body.

GLOSSARY—continued

hypertension—High blood pressure. Diagnosed when at least two blood pressure readings on separate occasions are 140/90 mm Hg or higher.

hypertensive crisis—A condition characterized by extremely high blood pressure levels (diastolic pressure above 120 mm Hg). Occurs in about 1% of people with hypertension.

hypotension—Low blood pressure. Can cause dizziness or light-headedness.

insulin—A hormone that controls the manufacture of glucose by the liver and permits muscle and fat cells to remove glucose from the blood. High blood insulin levels can cause hypertension.

intermittent claudication—Pain in the leg muscles caused by an inadequate supply of oxygen and blood to the legs. Most often occurs with walking.

intracerebral hemorrhage—Leakage of blood from a damaged blood vessel into tissues deep within the brain.

ischemia—A lack of oxygen due to a decrease in blood supply to a body organ or tissue.

ischemic cascade—A chain of chemical reactions, occurring during an ischemic stroke, that leads to a buildup of toxins and further cell destruction. Also called glutamate cascade.

ischemic stroke—A stroke resulting from the blockage of an artery supplying blood to the brain.

isolated systolic hypertension—A systolic blood pressure of 140 mm Hg or higher along with a diastolic blood pressure under 90 mm Hg. Associated with an increased risk of strokes, coronary heart disease, and kidney disease.

J-curve phenomenon—Refers to the relationship between the risk of a heart attack and blood pressure. The curve shows that those with the highest and lowest blood pressure levels are more likely to die of a heart attack than those with an intermediate blood pressure level. Many experts question whether the J-curve phenomenon actually exists.

kidneys—A pair of organs, located on the left and right sides of the abdomen, that remove waste products and excess water from the blood and produce urine.

lacunar stroke—A stroke that occurs when the tiny branches at the end of arteries in the brain become completely blocked by small emboli or atherosclerotic plaque.

left ventricular hypertrophy—A thickening of the muscular wall of the left ventricle that occurs when it must work harder to pump blood. Common in people with hypertension.

limb contracture—Consistent tightening of ligaments and tendons in the limbs.

limbic system—A group of structures in the brain responsible for primal urges and powerful emotions, such as hunger and terror, that help ensure self-preservation.

low density lipoprotein (LDL)—A particle that transports cholesterol in the bloodstream and is a major contributor to coronary heart disease. Its deposition in artery walls initiates plaque formation.

magnetic resonance angiography (MRA)—A technique for viewing the arteries in the neck, brain, or other organs. Similar to an MRI.

magnetic resonance imaging (MRI)—A test that employs magnetic fields and radio waves to generate a three-dimensional image of a part of the body, such as the brain.

metabolic syndrome—A group of findings, including obesity, hypertension, high triglyceride levels, low HDL cholesterol levels, and elevated blood glucose levels, that is caused by a genetic predisposition to insulin resistance and an accumulation of fat in the abdomen. Previously called insulin resistance syndrome or syndrome X.

motor cortex—A part of the frontal lobe of the brain. Damage to this area can result in weakness or paralysis on the opposite side of the body.

neuron—Nerve cell.

nitric oxide—A substance secreted by cells lining the walls of blood vessels that causes arteries to dilate by relaxing smooth muscle cells.

norepinephrine—A hormone that increases blood pressure in response to stress.

occipital lobe—An area of the brain at the back of the skull that is dedicated to the perception and interpretation of visual data from the eyes.

orthostatic hypotension—Abrupt drop in blood pressure on standing that causes dizziness or light-headedness. A side effect of many antihypertensive medications.

parathyroid hormone—A hormone that regulates calcium metabolism. It dilates small arteries that may play a role in the control of blood pressure.

parietal lobe—An area of the brain behind the frontal lobe that receives and interprets sensory signals from all parts of the body.

peripheral-acting adrenergic antagonists—Drugs that reduce resistance to blood flow in small arteries.

peripheral vascular disease—A narrowing of the arteries in the extremities, usually the legs. Most often due to atherosclerosis.

pheochromocytoma—A tumor in the adrenal gland that secretes large amounts of epinephrine or norepinephrine. Can lead to hypertension.

plaque—An accumulation of cholesterol, smooth muscle cells, fibrous proteins, and calcium in artery walls.

potassium—A mineral found mainly in fruits and vegetables. Increased intake helps lower blood pressure.

prehypertension—A new term used to describe individuals with systolic blood pressures between 120 and 139 mm Hg or diastolic blood pressures between 80 and 89 mm Hg. These individuals are at high risk for developing hypertension.

primary hypertension—Hypertension likely related to a poor diet, excess weight, high sodium intake, or physical inactivity. Affects 90% to 95% of people with hypertension.

pulse pressure—The difference between systolic and diastolic blood pressures. Reflects the stiffness of arteries.

renin—An enzyme produced by cells in the kidney that converts angiotensinogen to angiotensin I.

renovascular hypertension—A type of hypertension caused by a reduction in blood flow to the kidneys.

retinopathy—Damage to the retina of the eye caused by changes in the tiny blood vessels that supply the retina. The leading cause of blindness in U.S. adults.

salt—Another term for sodium chloride (table salt). One teaspoon of salt contains 2,400 mg of sodium.

secondary hypertension—Hypertension caused by another health condition or a medication. Responsible for less than 5% of cases of hypertension.

sodium—A mineral found mostly in processed foods, including salted snacks, canned soups, luncheon meats, and frozen dinners. In general, diets high in sodium cause blood pressure to rise. Sodium intake should be limited to no more than 2,400 mg per day.

sphygmomanometer—An instrument used to measure blood pressure. Consists of an inflating bulb, inflatable cuff, and gauge.

spiral computed tomography (CT) scanning—An imaging method in which an iodine-based dye is injected into the patient and a rapid CT scan is performed through the region of interest. Computer-based software then shows images of the blood vessels that fill with dye.

stent—A wire mesh tube that is inserted into an artery to help keep it open.

stroke—A sudden reduction in or loss of brain function that occurs when an artery supplying blood to a portion of the brain becomes blocked or ruptures. Neurons in the affected area are starved of the oxygen and nutrients they need to function properly.

subarachnoid hemorrhage—Leakage of blood into the space between the brain and the arachnoid membrane, the middle of three membranes that envelop the brain. Most commonly results from trauma or a ruptured aneurysm.

systolic blood pressure—The upper number in a blood pressure reading. Represents pressure in the arteries when the heart is pumping blood to the rest of the body.

temporal lobe—An area of the brain at ear level underneath the parietal and frontal lobes that is dedicated to auditory perception and storage of memories.

thrombolytic drugs—Medications that dissolve blood clots.

thrombus—A blood clot. The plural form is thrombi.

transient ischemic attack (TIA)—Short-lived neurological deficits caused by insufficient blood flow to the brain. Most episodes subside within 5 to 20 minutes.

triglyceride—A lipid (fat) in the bloodstream. Elevated levels are associated with an increased risk of coronary heart disease.

vasospasm—A constriction of blood vessels in the brain that is likely to occur in the first two weeks after a subarachnoid hemorrhage.

vertebral arteries—Blood vessels that run up the back of the neck, parallel to the spine, and carry blood to the brain stem and rear third of the brain.

white coat hypertension—High blood pressure readings that are present only when the patient's blood pressure is recorded by a physician or in a medical environment. Blood pressure is normal when taken at home by the patient, family members, or friends.

HEALTH INFORMATION ORGANIZATIONS AND SUPPORT GROUPS

American College of Cardiology
9111 Old Georgetown Rd.
Bethesda, MD 20814-1699
☎ 800-253-4636/301-897-5400
www.acc.org

Professional medical society and teaching institution that provides professional education, promotes research, offers leadership in the development of standards and guidelines, and forms health care policy.

American Heart Association
7272 Greenville Ave.
Dallas, TX 75231
☎ 800-242-8721
www.americanheart.org

National health organization that provides information and public education programs on all aspects of heart disease. Check for local chapters.

The American Occupational Therapy Association
4720 Montgomery Lane
P.O. Box 31220
Bethesda, MD 20824-1220
☎ 301-652-2682
800-377-8555 (TDD)
www.aota.org

Provides a consumer tip sheet and information about occupational therapy services for people recovering from a stroke and their families. Also provides contact information for state associations to aid in therapist referrals.

American Physical Therapy Association
1111 N. Fairfax St.
Alexandria, VA 22314-1488
☎ 800-999-APTA/703-684-APTA
www.apta.org

National professional organization for physical therapists (PTs) that provides referrals to state PT associations.

American Society of Hypertension
148 Madison Ave., 5th Fl.
New York, NY 10016
☎ 212-696-9099
www.ash-us.org

Largest U.S. organization dedicated exclusively to hypertension and related cardiovascular disease. Organizes and conducts educational programs to promote the development of treatments for hypertension.

American Speech-Language-Hearing Association
10801 Rockville Pike
Rockville, MD 20852
☎ 800-638-8255
www.asha.org

Toll-free help line gives information on communication disorders and referrals to speech-language pathologists and audiologists around the country.

American Stroke Association
7272 Greenville Ave.
Dallas, TX 75231
☎ 888-4-STROKE
800-553-6321 ("Warmline")
www.strokeassociation.org

A division of the American Heart Association; provides referrals to community stroke groups and information and peer counseling to survivors and caregivers. Call the "Warmline" to subscribe to their magazine, *Stroke Connection.*

HeartInfo.org—The Heart Information Network
26 Main St., 3rd Fl.
Chatham, NJ 09728
www.heartinfo.org

Educational Web site providing the latest news, advice, and self-help tools for the prevention, diagnosis, and treatment of cardiovascular disease.

Mended Hearts, Inc.
7272 Greenville Ave.
Dallas, TX 75231-4596
☎ 888-HEART-99/214-706-1442
www.mendedhearts.org

Support group for heart disease patients and their families. Call, write, or visit the Web site for information and to get in touch with other heart patients in your area.

National Aphasia Association
29 John St., #1103
New York, NY 10038
☎ 800-922-4622
www.aphasia.org

Provides educational material, a newsletter, a directory of community support groups, and a national network of volunteers who can discuss professional and social resources in their areas.

National Heart, Lung, and Blood Institute Information Center
P.O. Box 30105
Bethesda, MD 20824-0105
☎ 800-575-WELL/301-592-8573
www.nhlbi.nih.gov/health/infoctr/index.htm

Branch of the National Institutes of Health that provides written information on all heart-related issues.

National Institute of Neurological Disorders and Stroke
P.O. Box 5801
Bethesda, MD 20824
☎ 800-352-9424
www.ninds.nih.gov

Leading supporter of neurological research in the United States. Provides publications about neurological disorders and a list of voluntary health agencies.

National Rehabilitation Information Center
4200 Forbes Blvd., Ste. 202
Lanham, MD 20706
☎ 800-346-2742/301-459-5900
www.naric.com

National library providing information on rehabilitation and disability, including independent living, employment, medical rehabilitation, and legislation. Makes referrals to community rehabilitation centers.

National Stroke Association
9707 E. Easter Lane
Englewood, CO 80112
☎ 800-STROKES/303-649-9299
www.stroke.org

National nonprofit organization devoting 100% of its resources to stroke. Provides education, services, and community-based activities in stroke prevention, treatment, rehabilitation, and recovery.

LEADING HOSPITALS

U.S. News & World Report and the National Opinion Research Center, a social-science research group at the University of Chicago, recently conducted their 14th annual nationwide survey of 8,160 physicians in 17 medical specialties. The doctors nominated up to five hospitals they consider best from among 6,003 U.S. hospitals. These are the current lists of the best hospitals for neurology and cardiology, as determined by the doctors' recommendations from 2001, 2002, and 2003; federal data on death rates; and factual data regarding quality indicators, such as the ratio of registered nurses to patients and the use of advanced technology. Since the results reflect the doctors' opinions, however, they are, to some degree, subjective. Any institution listed is considered a leading center, and the rankings do not imply that other hospitals cannot or do not deliver excellent care.

NEUROLOGY AND NEUROSURGERY HOSPITALS

1. **Mayo Clinic**
   Rochester, MN
   ☎ 507-284-2511
   www.mayoclinic.org

2. **Massachusetts General Hospital**
   Boston, MA
   ☎ 617-726-2000
   www.mgh.harvard.edu

3. **Johns Hopkins Hospital**
   Baltimore, MD
   ☎ 800-507-9952/410-955-5000
   www.hopkinsmedicine.org

4. **New York-Presbyterian Hospital**
   New York, NY
   ☎ 212-305-2500
   www.nyp.org

5. **University of California, San Francisco Medical Center**
   San Francisco, CA
   ☎ 888-689-UCSF/415-476-1000
   www.ucsfhealth.org

6. **Cleveland Clinic**
   Cleveland, OH
   ☎ 800-223-2273/216-444-2200
   www.clevelandclinic.org

7. **Barnes-Jewish Hospital**
   St. Louis, MO
   ☎ 314-747-3000
   www.barnesjewish.org

8. **University of California, Los Angeles Medical Center**
   Los Angeles, CA
   ☎ 800-825-2631/310-825-9111
   www.healthcare.ucla.edu

9. **Hospital of the University of Pennsylvania**
   Philadelphia, PA
   ☎ 800-789-PENN/215-662-4000
   www.pennhealth.com/upmc

10. **St. Joseph's Hospital and Medical Center**
    Phoenix, AZ
    ☎ 602-406-3000
    www.ichosestjoes.com

CARDIOLOGY AND HEART SURGERY HOSPITALS

1. **Cleveland Clinic**
   Cleveland, OH
   ☎ 800-223-2273/216-444-2200
   www.clevelandclinic.org

2. **Mayo Clinic**
   Rochester, MN
   ☎ 507-284-2511
   www.mayoclinic.org

3. **Brigham and Women's Hospital**
   Boston, MA
   ☎ 617-732-5500
   www.brighamandwomens.org

4. **Duke University Medical Center**
   Durham, NC
   ☎ 919-684-8111
   www.mc.duke.edu

5. **Massachusetts General Hospital**
   Boston, MA
   ☎ 617-726-2000
   www.mgh.harvard.edu

6. **Johns Hopkins Hospital**
   Baltimore, MD
   ☎ 800-507-9952/410-955-5000
   www.hopkinsmedicine.org

7. **Emory University Hospital**
   Atlanta, GA
   ☎ 800-75-EMORY/404-778-7777
   www.emoryhealthcare.org

8. **Texas Heart Institute at St. Luke's Episcopal Hospital**
   Houston, TX
   ☎ 800-292-2221
   www.texasheartinstitute.org

9. **Stanford Hospital and Clinics**
   Stanford, CA
   ☎ 650-723-4000
   www.stanfordhospital.com

10. **Barnes-Jewish Hospital**
    St. Louis, MO
    ☎ 314-747-3000
    www.barnesjewish.org

LOWERING BLOOD PRESSURE FOR STROKE PREVENTION

Doctors have long known that blood pressure control can reduce the risk of a first stroke. Now, more recent evidence demonstrates that lowering blood pressure in those who have already had a stroke can help prevent future strokes, even in people without hypertension. In the article reprinted here from *The American Journal of Cardiology,* John Chalmers, M.D., of the University of Sydney in Australia, reviews the evidence for antihypertensive therapy for prevention of second strokes. Most important, he reviews the results of a landmark study—the Perindopril Protection Against Recurrent Stroke Study (PROGRESS)—which showed that antihypertensive therapy effectively reduced the risk of strokes and heart attacks in people who previously had a stroke or transient ischemic attack (TIA).

In PROGRESS, 6,105 people who had a nondisabling stroke or TIA in the past five years were randomized to receive an active treatment or a placebo. The active treatment was the ACE inhibitor perindopril (Aceon), either alone or in combination with the diuretic indapamide (Lozol). About half of the people had hypertension and half did not. Participants were told to continue taking their current treatments, such as antiplatelet therapy and other antihypertensive drugs.

After four years, patients in the active-treatment group were 24% less likely to have had an ischemic stroke and 50% less likely to have had a hemorrhagic stroke than those taking the placebo. The reduction in stroke risk occurred regardless of the patients' initial blood pressure levels. Overall, the patients were also 26% less likely to have a heart attack or stroke compared with the placebo group. However, these risk reductions occurred mainly in people receiving perindopril plus indapamide, rather than perindopril alone. The improved outcomes with combination therapy were likely the result of better blood pressure lowering with perindopril plus indapamide than with perindopril alone (a reduction of 12/5 vs. 5/3 mm Hg).

In people who have suffered a stroke or TIA, Dr. Chalmers recommends that antihypertensive therapy should begin on discharge from the hospital or at the first postdischarge doctor visit. But even people who have had a stroke or TIA years before can benefit from antihypertensive therapy, he writes. For the greatest benefit, antihypertensive therapy after a stroke or TIA should consist of an ACE inhibitor and diuretic.

Trials on Blood Pressure–Lowering and Secondary Stroke Prevention

John Chalmers, MD

The risk of stroke is strongly and persistently related to the usual level of both systolic blood pressure (SBP) and diastolic blood pressure (DBP). This relation holds for primary and secondary stroke, both ischemic and hemorrhagic. The Perindopril Protection Against Recurrent Stroke Study (PROGRESS) has now provided definitive evidence that lowering the blood pressure of patients with preexisting cerebrovascular disease (prior stroke or transient ischemic attack [TIA]) also reduces the incidence of secondary stroke. PROGRESS showed that a flexible blood pressure–lowering regimen involving an angiotensin-converting enzyme inhibitor (perindopril) and a diuretic (indapamide) reduces the incidence of stroke, major coronary events, and major vascular events by 28%, 26%, and 26%, respectively. These benefits were associated with an average reduction of 9.0 mm Hg (SBP) and 4.0 mm Hg (DBP). The 28% reduction in stroke incidence translated into a 24% reduction in ischemic stroke and a 50% reduction in hemorrhagic stroke. Combination therapy with perindopril and indapamide decreased blood pressure more effectively than did perindopril monotherapy (mean reduction of 12.3 mm Hg [SBP] and 5.0 mm Hg [DBP] vs 4.9 mm Hg [SBP] and 2.8 mm Hg [DBP], respectively) and was equally effective in reducing stroke risk in patients with and without hypertension. In conclusion, blood pressure–lowering therapy is now established as the most important measure for primary and secondary stroke prevention. Results of PROGRESS suggest that antihypertensive treatment with a combination of perindopril plus indapamide should now be routinely considered for all patients with previous stroke or TIA.

Am J Cardiol 2003;91(suppl):3G–8G

A landmark analysis of 9 prospective observational North American and European studies involving almost 420,000 individuals established that the risk of a primary stroke or coronary event is strongly and continuously related to diastolic blood pressure (DBP) level.[1] Within the range of DBP studied (approximately 70 mm Hg to 110 mm Hg), there was no evidence for a threshold level below which the risk of stroke or coronary artery disease would no longer correlate with DBP. Thus, for most people, lowering blood pressure should decrease their risk of vascular disease, regardless of whether they were typically classified as hypertensive or normotensive.

The association between stroke risk and blood pressure is not confined to these populations, because studies in Australia/New Zealand and Asia have revealed a correlation between systolic blood pressure (SBP) level and the risk of a primary stroke.[2] The relation was powerful for both hemorrhagic and ischemic stroke and predicted that a 10-mm Hg reduction in SBP would reduce the risk of a hemorrhagic stroke by 29% and of ischemic stroke by 25% in the Australia/New Zealand cohort, and by 41% and 35%, respectively, in the Asian cohort.[2]

PRIMARY PREVENTION OF STROKE

Because elevated blood pressure predisposes patients to a primary stroke or to coronary artery disease, a number of randomized, controlled clinical trials were initiated to investigate whether antihypertensive therapy could reduce these risks. A meta-analysis was conducted on 17 such trials, which together involved 47,667 patients treated predominantly with diuretic- and/or β-blocker–based regimens for about 5 years.[3] This overview found that a decrease of 5 to 6 mm Hg in DBP or 10 to 12 mm Hg in SBP over an average treatment period of 2 to 3 years conferred a 38% reduction in the incidence of primary stroke, with equivalent reductions in fatal and nonfatal strokes. Appropriate analysis of prospective epidemiologic studies indicated that a prolonged difference of 5 to 7.5 mm Hg in usual DBP would eventually be associated with differences of about 34% to 46% in the risk of stroke.[1] Thus, the trial evidence is consistent with the expectations from observational data.

The Blood Pressure Lowering Treatment Trialists' Collaboration has reported the effects of angiotensin-converting enzyme (ACE) inhibitors and calcium channel blockers on cardiovascular morbidity and mortality, including stroke.[4] These overviews revealed reductions in stroke risk of 30% (95% confidence interval, 15% to 43%) with ACE inhibitors and 39% (95% confidence interval, 15% to 56%) with calcium antagonists compared with placebo. Furthermore, in the trials comparing ACE inhibitor–based regimens with more traditional diuretic- or β-blocker–based regimens (Swedish Trial in Old Patients with Hypertension-2 [STOP-2][5] and UK Prospective Diabetes Study-Hypertension Diabetes Study [UKPDS-HDS][6,7]), these different classes of antihypertensive agents offered similar benefits in the prevention of stroke (Figure 1).

From the Institute for International Health, University of Sydney, Newton, Australia.

Address for reprints: John Chalmers, MD, Institute of International Health, University of Sydney, 144-146 Burren Street, Newton, NSW 2042 Australia. E-mail: chalmers@iih.usyd.edu.au.

0002-9149/03/$ – see front matter
doi:10.1016/S0002-9149(03)00226-1

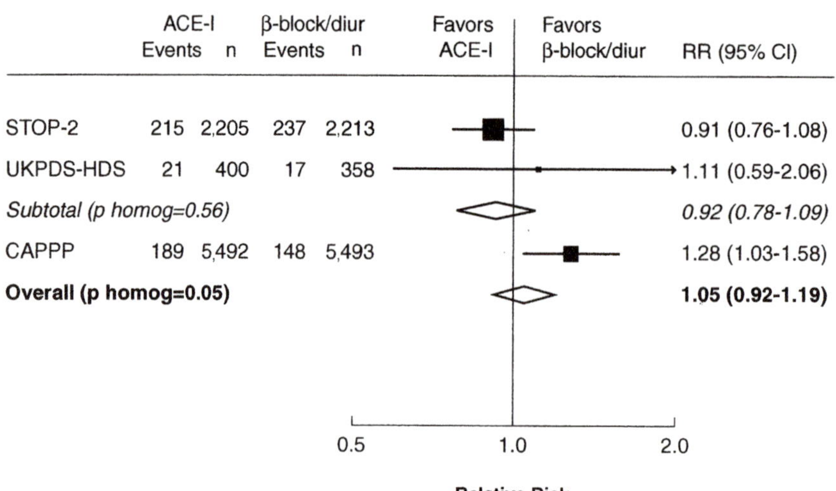

FIGURE 1. Comparative influence of ACE-inhibitor (ACE-I)–based therapy with diuretic (diur)- or β-blocker (β-block)–based therapy on stroke risk. CAPPP = Captopril Prevention Project; CI = confidence interval; p homog = p-value from χ^2 test for homogeneity; RR = relative risk; STOP-2 = Swedish Trial in Old Patients with Hypertension-2; UKPDS-HDS = UK Prospective Diabetes Study-Hypertension Diabetes Study. (Adapted with permission from *Lancet*.[4,10])

TABLE 1 The Beneficial Effect of Treatment with Ramipril on the Composite Outcome of Myocardial Infarction, Stroke, or Death from Cardiovascular Causes Overall and in Various Predefined Subgroups*

CVD Death, MI, or Stroke	HR	95% CI
Overall	0.78	0.70–0.86
History of CVD	0.78	0.71–0.87
No history of CVD	0.81	0.56–1.20
Diabetics	0.76	0.65–0.89
Nondiabetics	0.79	0.69–0.91
Hypertensive	0.75	0.65–0.87
Nonhypertensive	0.81	0.70–0.93

*Heart Outcomes Prevention Evaluation (HOPE) trial: ramipril vs placebo resulted in a 3-mm Hg reduction in systolic blood pressure.
Adapted with permission from *N Engl J Med*.[8]

THE HEART OUTCOMES PREVENTION EVALUATION TRIAL

The Heart Outcomes Prevention Evaluation (HOPE) trial results showed that the benefits of lowering blood pressure on the risk of stroke are not confined to patients with hypertension, but they also extend to individuals with blood pressure within the normotensive range.[8] HOPE was a randomized, double-blind, placebo-controlled study examining the effects of ramipril on major vascular events in high-risk patients. It enrolled 9,297 subjects ≥55 years of age with coronary or peripheral vascular disease, stroke, or diabetes plus ≥1 additional cardiovascular risk factor but with normal left ventricular function. Hypertension was not an inclusion criterion, and only 47.6% of patients were hypertensive. Patients were assigned to ramipril 10 mg or matching placebo for a mean of 5 years.

Compared with placebo, ramipril reduced the risk of stroke by 32% (p <0.001). Other benefits included reduction of risk for a primary cardiovascular event (cardiovascular death, stroke, or acute myocardial infarction) by 22% (p <0.001) and reduction of cardiovascular mortality by 26% (p <0.001) and of myocardial infarction by 20% (p <0.001). The beneficial effects of ramipril on the primary outcome were consistent across a range of subgroups examined (Table 1).[8]

SECONDARY PREVENTION OF STROKE

The value of antihypertensive therapy in primary stroke prevention is unequivocal. However, whether long-term lowering of blood pressure has a similar impact on stroke risk in patients who have sustained an a priori cerebrovascular event has been the subject of some controversy, which has only just been re-

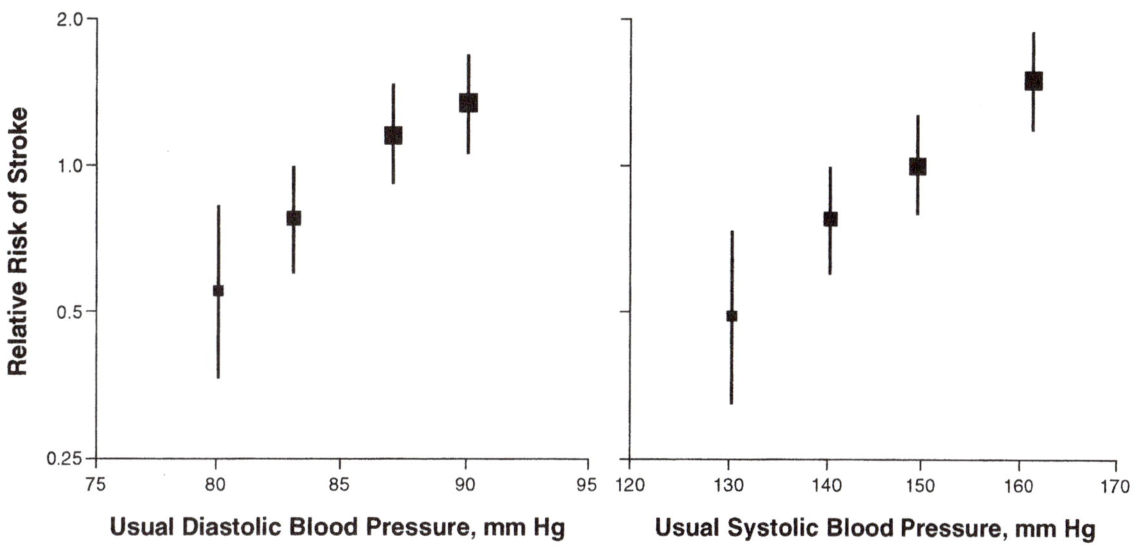

FIGURE 2. Relation between usual diastolic and systolic blood pressure and stroke in the United Kingdom Transient Ischaemic Attack (UK-TIA) aspirin trial. (Reprinted with permission from *BMJ*.[10])

solved. This is an important consideration because the risk of a second stroke or recurrent stroke is elevated substantially among individuals who have already experienced a first stroke or transient ischemic attack (TIA). A second stroke will add to the likelihood of death and disability, with corresponding implications on societal costs in health care provision to survivors.[9]

Strategies aimed at preventing secondary stroke have mainly been targeted toward patients who have sustained an a priori ischemic stroke. Until recently, there were no proven preventive treatments for patients with a history of intracerebral hemorrhage. Antiplatelet agents, such as aspirin and clopidogrel, reduce the relative risk of a recurrent ischemic stroke by approximately 20% compared with placebo and are now standard therapy for patients with previous stroke or TIA. Other therapies may be appropriate for selected individuals: anticoagulants are routinely used to decrease the stroke risk among patients with atrial fibrillation, and carotid endarterectomy may help to reduce the risk of recurrent ipsilateral stroke among patients with carotid stenosis. Because of limitations of current therapies, physicians have become increasingly interested in additional approaches to recurrent stroke prevention, such as antihypertensive therapy.

Perhaps the most compelling observational data supporting the importance of elevated blood pressure in increasing the risk of a secondary stroke come from a retrospective analysis of the United Kingdom Transient Ischemic Attack (UK-TIA) aspirin trial.[10] The 2,435 patients included in this analysis had a history of minor ischemic stroke or TIA. As seen in Figure 2,[10] direct and continuous relations were observed between stroke and both DBP and SBP. A 5-mm Hg reduction in usual DBP and a 10-mm Hg reduction in usual SBP were associated with 34% (SD ± 7%) and 28% (SD ± 8%) fewer strokes, respectively. There was no evidence to support the existence of a J-shaped curve.

PERINDOPRIL PROTECTION AGAINST RECURRENT STROKE STUDY

In 1997, a meta-analysis of 9 randomized, controlled, clinical trials was conducted to assess the effect of antihypertensive drugs on clinical outcomes in patients with prior stroke or TIA.[11] A 28% (95% confidence interval, 15% to 39%) reduction in the recurrence of fatal and nonfatal stroke was reported. Although this meta-analysis provided an initial indication that blood pressure–lowering therapy has a role in secondary stroke prevention in hypertensive subjects, it had several limitations. As a result, many questions on the absolute benefits of blood pressure–lowering therapy in patients who have already sustained a cerebrovascular event remained unanswered—such as its value in normotensive stroke survivors.

The Perindopril Protection Against Recurrent Stroke Study (PROGRESS) was designed to resolve uncertainties about the value of blood pressure–lowering therapy in secondary stroke prevention.[12] The main objective of PROGRESS was to determine the effects of a flexible antihypertensive regimen involving an ACE inhibitor (perindopril) and a diuretic (indapamide) on the risk of stroke and other major vascular events among hypertensive and nonhypertensive patients with preexisting cerebrovascular disease (defined as previous TIA or stroke).

PROGRESS was a randomized, double-blind, placebo-controlled trial conducted at 172 centers in Asia, Australasia, and Europe. Active treatment was with a flexible antihypertensive regimen based on perindopril 4 mg/day, with the addition of indapamide 2.5 mg/day at the discretion of the investigator—in addition to whatever other medication the patient was already taking. Perindopril was chosen as the ACE inhibitor because of the following: (1) it has a long duration of action, providing smooth 24-hour blood pressure control from a once-daily dose; (2) it has a minimal first-dose effect; and (3) it does not compromise cerebral blood flow. Indapamide was selected as add-on therapy because it has not been associated with deleterious changes in metabolic parameters, such as glucose metabolism,[13] and the combination of an ACE inhibitor plus indapamide has been shown to be efficacious in hypertensive patients.[14] Flexibility in the use of monotherapy versus combination therapy for each patient was intended to offset any reservations the investigators might have had about administering intensive antihypertensive therapy to patients with cerebrovascular disease and normal blood pressure. Follow-up evaluation continued for an average of 4 years.

Patients: To be eligible for PROGRESS, patients had to have had a nondisabling stroke or TIA in the past 5 years and no definite indication or contraindication for ACE inhibitor treatment. There were no blood pressure entry criteria, but it was recommended that hypertensive patients have their blood pressure controlled with drugs other than ACE inhibitors before entry into the trial. In addition, all patients were to be clinically stable for ≥2 weeks after their most recent cerebrovascular accident.

A total of 6,105 subjects entered the trial, of which 3,051 were randomized to active treatment (1,281 of 3,051 [42%] receiving perindopril alone and 1,770 of 3,051 [58%] receiving perindopril plus indapamide) and 3,054 to placebo.[15] The 2 treatment groups were well matched in all documented baseline characteristics: in both groups, the mean age was 64 years, 30% were women, 13% had diabetes, and 16% had documented coronary artery disease. With regard to blood pressure status at baseline, 48% were hypertensive, 50% were receiving antihypertensive medication, mean SBP was 147 mm Hg, and mean DBP was 86 mm Hg.

Blood pressure reductions: Active treatment with the perindopril-based regimen reduced blood pressure by a mean of 9.0 mm Hg (SBP) and 4.0 mm Hg (DBP) over placebo, a difference that was maintained throughout the entire follow-up period.[15] Placebo-adjusted blood pressure reductions were greater among patients on perindopril/indapamide combination therapy (12 mm Hg [SBP] and 5 mm Hg [DBP]) than among those on perindopril monotherapy (5 mm Hg [SBP] and 3 mm Hg [DBP]) and were similar between patients classified as hypertensive and nonhypertensive.

Reduction in stroke risk: Lowering blood pressure in the PROGRESS trial by just 9.0 mm Hg (SBP) and 4.0 mm Hg (DBP) with perindopril-based therapy decreased the risk of fatal or nonfatal secondary stroke (the primary trial outcome) by 28% versus placebo (95% confidence interval, 17% to 38%; $p < 0.0001$). The difference became apparent within the first year of treatment and widened as the study progressed, showing that the perindopril-based regimen had an early and persistent effect on stroke prevention (Figure 3). These benefits were achieved by the addition of perindopril-based therapy to the patient's existing medication, including antihypertensive drugs and antiplatelet agents for many patients with a history of ischemic stroke or TIA. The benefits of active treatment were apparent for all stroke subtypes, with the greatest reduction seen for intracranial hemorrhage (Figure 4).

For the patients receiving the combination of perindopril plus indapamide, blood pressure was reduced by a mean of 12.3 mm Hg (SBP) and 5.0 mm Hg (DBP). Among these patients, treatment reduced the secondary stroke risk by 43% (95% confidence interval, 30% to 54%). In contrast, the stroke risk for patients receiving perindopril alone (mean blood pressure reduction, 4.9 mm Hg [SBP] and 2.8 mm Hg [DBP]), and those receiving placebo was not significantly different. The greater reduction in stroke risk with the combination therapy compared with the monotherapy may be attributable to the greater blood pressure reduction achieved with the combination therapy.

Finally, comparison of stroke risk for all patients receiving active treatment showed reductions for hypertensive and nonhypertensive patients alike (p-value for homogeneity = 0.7),[15] indicating that lowering blood pressure offers benefits, regardless of the initial blood pressure level.

Reduction in risk of major vascular events: A secondary end point in PROGRESS was a composite of the following major vascular events: nonfatal stroke, nonfatal myocardial infarction, or death because of any vascular cause. Perindopril-based therapy lowered the risk of this composite end point by 26% (95% confidence interval, 16% to 34%) versus placebo, driven mainly by a pronounced reduction in the risk of nonfatal myocardial infarction (38% relative risk reduction; 95% confidence interval, 14% to 15%).[15] As with stroke, the risk of major vascular events was decreased more by perindopril plus indapamide combination therapy (40% relative risk reduction; 95% confidence interval, 29% to 49%) than by perindopril alone (4% relative risk reduction; 95% confidence interval, −15% to 20%).

The risk of major vascular events was also reduced in patients regardless of whether they were classified as hypertensive (29% relative risk reduction; 95% confidence interval, 16% to 40%) or nonhypertensive (24% relative risk reduction; 95% confidence interval, 9% to 37%) at baseline.

Safety and tolerability: Perindopril, with or without indapamide, was very well tolerated over the 4-year follow-up period.[15] The rates of premature discontinuation were similar between patients assigned active treatment and those assigned placebo (23% vs 21%, p = 0.02). More patients receiving perindopril-based therapy than placebo withdrew because of hypotension (2.1% vs 0.9%) and cough (2.2% vs 0.4%), common side effects of ACE inhibitors. The low rate of hypotension is reassuring because >50% of patients were deemed nonhypertensive at baseline. Discontinuation rates were broadly similar between hypertensive and nonhypertensive patients receiving active treatment (22% vs 25%).

0.20
0.15
0.10
0.05
0.00
Proportion with Event
Placebo
Active
28% risk reduction
95% CI 17-38%
P<0.0001
0
1
2
3
4
Years

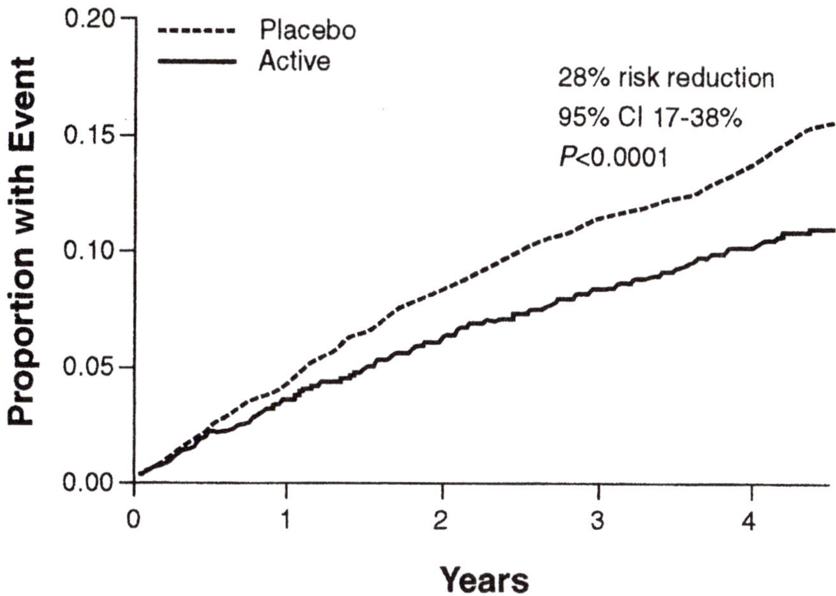

FIGURE 3. Stroke risk reduction (all participants). Cumulative incidence of stroke among patients assigned active treatment (perindopril ± indapamide) and those assigned placebo in the Perindopril Protection Against Recurrent Stroke Study (PROGRESS). CI = confidence interval. (Reprinted with permission from *Lancet*.[15])

Strokes
Active Placebo
Favors Active
Favors Placebo
Risk Reduction (95% CI)
Fatal/Disabling 123 181 33% (15% - 46%)
Other Stroke 201 262 24% (9% - 37%)
Cerebral Infarction 246 319 24% (10% - 35%)
Cerebral Hemorrhage 37 74 50% (26% - 67%)
Stroke Type Unknown 42 51 18% (-24% - 45%)
Total 307 420 28% (17% - 38%)
0.5
1.0
2.0
Hazard Ratio

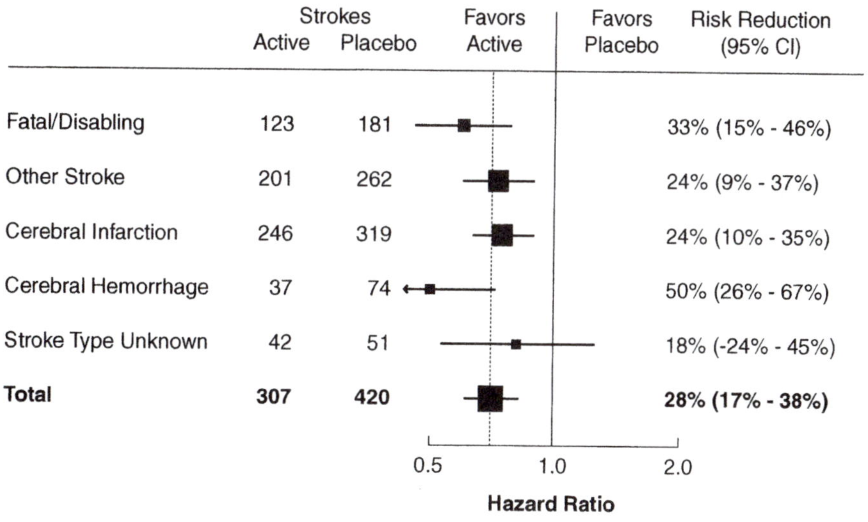

FIGURE 4. Stroke severity and subtype: effects of active treatment (perindopril ± indapamide) on stroke subtypes in the Perindopril Protection Against Recurrent Stroke Study (PROGRESS). CI = confidence interval. (Adapted with permission from *Lancet*.[15])

PERINDOPRIL PROTECTION AGAINST RECURRENT STROKE STUDY TREATMENT IMPLICATIONS

The PROGRESS results suggest that virtually all patients with previous stroke can benefit from blood pressure–lowering therapy with the study drugs. They indicate that 1 fatal or nonfatal vascular event could be prevented for every 11 patients treated with perindopril plus indapamide for 5 years. Given the large number of patients who have minor strokes or TIAs and the absolute benefit that can be achieved, the clinical implications of the PROGRESS findings are immense.

For patients with acute stroke, antihypertensive therapy should be initiated once the patient has been stabilized (not during the acute phase after a stroke, when cerebral autoregulatory mechanisms are disturbed). In practical terms, this would mean initiating treatment at the time of discharge or at the first postdischarge visit. Patients also appear to benefit from therapy, even if several years have elapsed from the time of the first cerebrovascular event. The physician at their next consultation should start such patients on treatment.

Treatment may commence with perindopril monotherapy; however, the PROGRESS results indicate that the combination of perindopril and indapamide offers the greatest benefit. Therefore, the aim should be to move patients onto combination therapy as soon as possible.

CONCLUSIONS

PROGRESS has provided the first definitive evidence that lowering blood pressure using a flexible, perindopril-based regimen reduces the risk of recurrent stroke in patients with a history of stroke or TIA.[15] The PROGRESS trial shows that the risk of all major types of stroke was lowered, with the greatest reduction seen for intracranial hemorrhage. The PROGRESS results support blood pressure–lowering therapy for secondary stroke prevention, not only for patients with hypertension, but also for nonhypertensive individuals. Perindopril-based therapy also reduced the overall risk of major vascular events (nonfatal stroke, nonfatal myocardial infarction, or death caused by any vascular cause), with a particularly strong impact on nonfatal myocardial infarction. Widespread implementation of PROGRESS treatment would avert vast numbers of stroke worldwide each year.

1. MacMahon S, Peto R, Cutler J, Collins R, Sorlie P, Neaton J, Abbott R, Godwin J, Dyer A, Stamler J. Blood pressure, stroke, and coronary heart disease: Part 1. Prolonged differences in blood pressure: prospective observational studies corrected for the regression dilution bias. *Lancet* 1990;335:765–774.
2. Eastern Stroke and Coronary Heart Disease Collaborative Research Group. Blood pressure, cholesterol, and stroke in Eastern Asia. *Lancet* 1998;352:1801–1807.
3. MacMahon S, Rodgers A. Blood pressure, antihypertensive treatment and stroke risk. *J Hypertens* 1994;12(suppl 10):S5–S14.
4. Neal B, MacMahon S, Chapman N. Effects of ACE inhibitors, calcium antagonists, and other blood-pressure-lowering drugs: results of prospectively designed overviews of randomised trials: Blood Pressure Lowering Treatment Trialists' Collaboration. *Lancet* 2000;356:1955–1964.
5. Hansson L, Lindholm LH, Ekbom T, Dahlöf B, Lanke J, Schersten B, Wester PO, Hedner T, de Faire U. Randomised trial of old and new antihypertensive drugs in elderly patients: cardiovascular mortality and morbidity the Swedish Trial in Old Patients with Hypertension-2 study. *Lancet* 1999;354:1751–1756.
6. Tight blood pressure control and risk of macrovascular and microvascular complications in type 2 diabetes: UKPDS 38, UK Prospective Diabetes Study Group. *BMJ* 1998;317:703–713.
7. Kannel WB, Wolf PA, Benjamin EJ, Levy D. Prevalence, incidence, prognosis, and predisposing conditions for atrial fibrillation: population-based estimates. *Am J Cardiol* 1998;82(suppl):2N–9N.
8. Yusuf S, Sleight P, Pogue J, Bosch J, Davies R, Dagenais G, et al. for the Heart Outcomes Prevention Evaluation Study Investigators. Effects of an angiotensin-converting-enzyme inhibitor, ramipril, on cardiovascular events in high-risk patients. *N Engl J Med* 2000;342:145–153.
9. Hankey GJ, Warlow CP. Treatment and secondary prevention of stroke: evidence, costs, and effects on individuals and populations. *Lancet* 1999;354: 1457–1463.
10. Rodgers A, MacMahon S, Gamble G, Slattery J, Sandercock P, Warlow C. Blood pressure and risk of stroke in patients with cerebrovascular disease: the United Kingdom Transient Ischaemic Attack Collaborative Group. *BMJ* 1996; 313:147.
11. Gueyffier F, Boissel JP, Boutitie F, Pocock S, Coope J, Cutler J, Ekbom T, Fagard R, Friedman L, Kerlikowske K, et al. Effect of antihypertensive treatment in patients having already suffered from stroke: gathering the evidence. The INDANA (INdividual Data ANalysis of Antihypertensive intervention trials) Project Collaborators. *Stroke* 1997;28:2557–2562.
12. Blood pressure lowering for the secondary prevention of stroke: rationale and design for PROGRESS. PROGRESS Management Committee: Perindopril Protection Against Recurrent Stroke Study. *J Hypertens Suppl* 1996;14(suppl): S41–S45; discussion S45–S46.
13. Weidmann P, de Courten M, Ferrari P, Bohlen L. Serum lipoproteins during treatment with antihypertensive drugs. *J Cardiovasc Pharmacol* 1993;22(suppl 6):S98–S105.
14. Matheson AJ, Cheer SM, Goa KL. Perindopril/indapamide 2/0.625 mg/day: a review of its place in the management of hypertension. *Drugs* 2001;61:1211–1229.
15. Randomised trial of a perindopril-based blood-pressure-lowering regimen among 6,105 individuals with previous stroke or transient ischaemic attack. *Lancet* 2001;358:1033–1041.

NOTES

NOTES

NOTES

ISBN 0-929661-94-X
ISSN 1542-1724
Fifth Printing
Printed in the United States of America

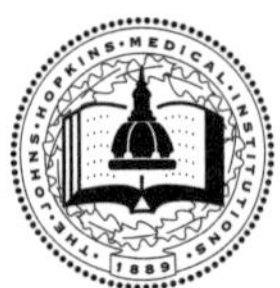

The Johns Hopkins White Papers are published yearly by Medletter Associates, Inc.

Visit our Web site for information on Johns Hopkins Health After 50 publications, which include White Papers on specific disorders, home medical encyclopedias, consumer reference guides to drugs and medical tests, and our monthly newsletter *The Johns Hopkins Medical Letter: Health After 50.*
www.HopkinsAfter50.com

The 2004 White Papers

64B60M

Take Control of Your Medical Condition

Visit us online at www.HopkinsAfter50.com

YES, I've placed a check mark next to the White Paper(s) I'd like to receive for $24.95 each. Annual updates on each subject that I have chosen will be offered to me by announcement card. I need do nothing if I want the update to be sent to me automatically. If I do not want it, I will return the announcement card marked "cancel." I may cancel at any time. (Please add $2.95 for domestic, $4.95 for Canadian, and $15.00 for foreign orders to your total to cover shipping and handling.) (Florida residents add sales tax.)

✔ Please put a check mark next to the White Paper(s) you wish to order.

- 001040 ❑ Arthritis $24.95
- 003046 ❑ Coronary Heart Disease $24.95
- 004044 ❑ Depression and Anxiety $24.95
- 005041 ❑ Diabetes $24.95
- 006049 ❑ Hypertension and Stroke $24.95
- 007047 ❑ Nutrition and Weight Control for Longevity $24.95
- 008045 ❑ Prostate Disorders $24.95
- 010041 ❑ Digestive Disorders $24.95
- 011049 ❑ Vision $24.95
- 012047 ❑ Back Pain & Osteoporosis $24.95
- 015040 ❑ Memory $24.95
- 019042 ❑ Lung Disorders $24.95
- 020040 ❑ Heart Attack Prevention $24.95

METHOD OF PAYMENT: (U.S. funds only) ❑ VISA ❑ Check Enclosed ❑ MasterCard ❑ Bill Me

Name

Address

City State Zip

Credit Card # Exp. Date

Signature Date

Money Back Guarantee: If for any reason, you are not satisfied after receipt of your publications, return your purchase within 30 days for a full refund.

Johns
Hopkins
White Papers

Fold along this line and tape closed

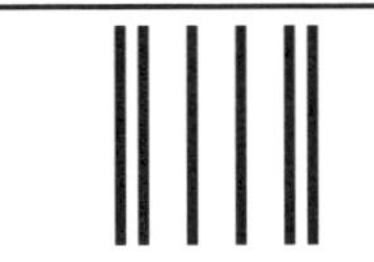

NO POSTAGE
NECESSARY
IF MAILED
IN THE
UNITED STATES

BUSINESS REPLY MAIL
FIRST-CLASS MAIL PERMIT NO. 86 FLAGLER BEACH FL

POSTAGE WILL BE PAID BY ADDRESSEE

THE JOHNS HOPKINS WHITE PAPERS
PO BOX 420083
PALM COAST FL 32142-9264

Johns
Hopkins
White Papers

Fold along this line and tape closed

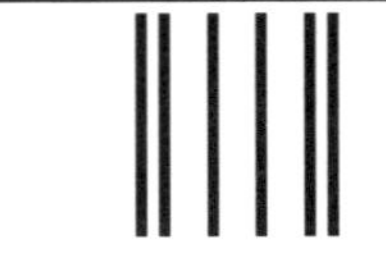

NO POSTAGE
NECESSARY
IF MAILED
IN THE
UNITED STATES

BUSINESS REPLY MAIL
FIRST-CLASS MAIL PERMIT NO. 86 FLAGLER BEACH FL

POSTAGE WILL BE PAID BY ADDRESSEE

THE JOHNS HOPKINS WHITE PAPERS
PO BOX 420083
PALM COAST FL 32142-9264

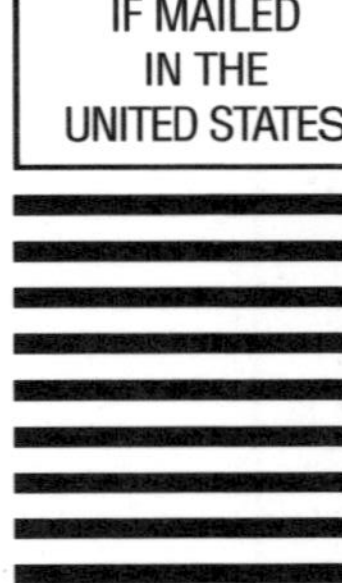

2004 WHITE PAPER TITLES

ARTHRITIS 2004 - Covers three common forms of arthritis - osteoarthritis, rheumatoid arthritis, and gout - as well as two other rheumatic diseases: fibromyalgia syndrome and bursitis.

CORONARY HEART DISEASE 2004 - Discusses four problems resulting from coronary heart disease: heart attacks, angina, cardiac arrhythmias, and heart failure.

DEPRESSION and ANXIETY 2004 - Includes major depression, dysthymia, atypical depression, bipolar disorder, seasonal affective disorder, panic disorder, generalized anxiety disorder, obsessive-compulsive disorder, post-traumatic stress disorder, and phobic disorders.

DIABETES 2004 - Shows you how to manage your diabetes and avoid complications such as foot problems and vision changes. Reviews the latest tools for monitoring your blood glucose and the newest medications for controlling it.

DIGESTIVE DISORDERS 2004 - Covers gastroesophageal reflux disease, peptic ulcers, dysphagia, achalasia, Barrett's esophagus, esophageal spasm and stricture, gastritis, gallstones, diarrhea, constipation, Crohn's disease, ulcerative colitis, and colon cancer.

HYPERTENSION and STROKE 2004 - Explains how to treat your high blood pressure and prevent it from harming your health. Also covers the two forms of stroke: ischemic stroke and hemorrhagic stroke.

BACK PAIN and OSTEOPOROSIS 2004 - Addresses back pain due to sprains, strains, and spasms; degenerative changes of the spinal bones and disks; disk herniation; and spinal stenosis. Also covers osteoporosis, a common cause of fractures in the spine and hip.

LUNG DISORDERS 2004 - Includes information on emphysema and chronic bronchitis (together referred to as chronic obstructive pulmonary disease or COPD), asthma, pneumonia, tuberculosis, lung cancer, and sleep apnea.

MEMORY 2004 - Tells you how to keep your memory sharp as you get older, and how to recognize the symptoms of age-associated memory impairment, mild cognitive impairment, and illnesses such as Alzheimer's disease and vascular dementia.

NUTRITION and WEIGHT CONTROL for LONGEVITY 2004 - Gives you the information you need to eat a healthy diet and keep your weight under control. Also explains what to do when the pounds just don't seem to budge.

PROSTATE DISORDERS 2004 - Helps you decide among the various treatment options for prostate cancer, benign prostatic hyperplasia, and prostatitis.

VISION 2004 - Reviews the current knowledge on cataracts, glaucoma, age-related macular degeneration, and diabetic retinopathy. Also discusses ways to cope with low vision.

HEART ATTACK PREVENTION 2004 - Provides up-to-date strategies for preventing a first heart attack, including identifying possible risk factors, the latest screening tests, risk-reducing lifestyle measures, and medications for controlling cholesterol.

9780929661940
HYPERTENSION AND STROKE